PRAISE FOR Leo F. Armbrust

"A powerful, meaningful work, *Only The Wounded May Serve*, is an inspirational gift to those of deep spirituality as well as a guide to practical, joyful living. It is an everyday understanding of one who has personally experienced life's depth and breadth, joy and pain, love and fear in his own life and the lives of others and thus can write so eloquently about it. Make no mistake: this work will ground you in living the good life in this ever-changing world."

- *Donna Tiernan Mahoney, Doctor of*

"I have known Leo for more th   during which he has been a valuable resource to me both personally and professionally. I have witnessed firsthand his ability to motivate and teach others important lessons for life; this book is but one example. I am proud to call him a friend."

- *Jimmy Johnson, NFL Analyst, Fox Sports*

"I've had the honor and privilege to be Leo's friend for the past twelve years. In his book, Leo draws on his personal, vocational, and professional experiences to share his insight into the human experience. More specifically, he challenges the reader to look within him/herself and explore essential elements of human existence and in turn, encourages a connection with the soul."

- *Dr. Adam Iglesias, Clinical Psychologist*

"Leo Armbrust is the Einstein of inspirational attainment and triumph in his beautifully written book."

- *Marti Huizenga*

"Now I understand why the nation's top football teams wanted Leo to counsel their players and sought his advice on issues far beyond tackling or touchdowns. This book provides a well-written road map for a healthy life — a triumph of both writing style and genuine storytelling."

- *Dave Hyde, Sports Columnist, South Florida Sun Sentinel*

"I have personally known Leo for thirty years; he is a dynamic life coach and speaker. He has helped me in so many ways with my professional and personal life with his guidance."

- *Bucky Dent, Former New York Yankee Shortstop and Manager*

"Leo is an entertaining speaker with a positive motivational message of importance and significance that appeals to all audiences. Bringing Leo to your group will be the highlight of your educational season..."

- *Dan Radakovich, Athletic Director, Clemson University*

ONLY THE WOUNDED MAY SERVE

"Father Leo has been a man of faith, community, and charity his entire life. Brilliant communicator from the lectern."

- *Thomas Hollywood Henderson, Former NFL Player*

"Leo Armbrust has spent his entire adult life in the service of others. He is an incredible communicator and a man of insight. Above all, Leo is a man that I'm proud to call my friend."

- *Kevin O'Neill, Athletic Trainer, NCAA & NFL*

"I have known Leo Armbrust for almost forty years. There is no finer motivational speaker; he is without peer. His message is clear, succinct, sprinkled with humor, and easily understood by all. He is truly a gifted individual."

- *Walter N. Colbath, Former Chief Judge, 15th Judicial Circuit of Florida*

"From 1991 until this day, whenever I see Fr. Leo anywhere, I ask him to 'Bless me, Father!' He was always there for me on game day at the U, but I'm also speaking of when I was in the NFL, I'd have a preseason game versus the Dolphins, and I would hug him and drop down to one knee and ask him to bless me. A real man of the world and always a friend!"

- *Warren Sapp, University of Miami (1991-1994), UM and NFL Hall of Famer*

"Leo has been our friend for many years. We have experienced firsthand the positive impact he has on the people around him. Leo has a true gift and ability to motivate, communicate, and provide the insight and guidance that can help all of us in our daily lives."

- *Rob and Sheila Chudzinski*

"I've known Leo for over three decades. He is a true mentor who has helped guide me through life's many challenges. His compassion is overwhelming and his understanding of the human spirit immense. From troubled teens to octogenarians, Leo seamlessly connects with everyone he meets."

- *David R. Heffernan, Esq., KAIRE & HEFFERNAN, LLC*

"From the football field to the political arena, Leo Armbrust has inspired so many of us with his passion, his optimism, and his wit. He can motivate anyone of any faith with his powerful communication style — and has a proven track record of doing so."

- *Dave Aronberg, State Attorney for Palm Beach County*

ONLY THE WOUNDED MAY SERVE

"Father Leo represents one of my most enduring and special relationships, going on more than thirty years now. His warmth, understanding, and insight are unique. He's one of those people who makes you think, appreciate, and do more to be a better person. I trust him with any matter of my personal life and cherish his advice. Father Leo's impact on my family extends to my young daughter. We proudly display his gift, a painting of the Annunciation, in her room. The accompanying letter is carefully tucked away in her closet to be saved for always. Writing this made me think: *I should turn to him more often and lean on him even more!*"

- *Suzy Kolber, ESPN Host/Reporter*

"On a personal level, may I just say that I'm proud to count Leo as a true friend."

- *Ron Sellers, Former FSU All-American & NFL Player*

"The time has come and I am so grateful that the dream has become a reality. Leo is one of the best communicators I have ever known. His book has the ability to guide us, to teach us, and immerse us into the most profound truths of life in a way that only he does."

- *Rev. Mario Castañeda, Founder of "Tu Palabra Hoy," an international preaching ministry, and Pastor of St. John Fisher Catholic Church*

Leo Armbrust

COVER ART

The fame of this powerful statue — named by scholars as "The Atlas" (or Bound Prisoner) — is due above all to its unfinished state. It is one of the finest examples of Michelangelo's habitual working practice, referred to as "non-finito" (or incomplete), a magnificent illustration of the difficulty of the artist in carving out the figure from the block of marble and is emblematic of the sruggle of man to free the spirit from matter.

This sculpture has been interpreted in many ways. As we view the sculpture in this stage of completion, it evokes the enormous strength of the creative concept as the man tries to free himself from the bonds and physical weight of the marble. The claim is that the artist deliberately left the work incomplete to represent the eternal struggle of human beings to free themselves from what holds them prisoner.

The sculpture is currently held in the Galleria dell'Accademia in Florence, Italy.

ONLY THE WOUNDED MAY SERVE
© 2016 By Leo F. Armbrust.

All rights reserved.

No part of this book may be used or reproduced in any manner whatsoever without written permission except in the case of brief quotations embodied in critical articles and reviews.

For information, email LEONIDAS, LLC. at author@leoarmbrust.cjom

Book may be purchased for educational, business, or sales promotional use.

For purchases and inquiries, please visit: www.leoarmbrust.com

ONLY THE WOUNDED MAY SERVE
PAPERBACK EDITION 2016

ONLY THE WOUNDED MAY SERVE
EBOOK EDITION 2016

Edited by Joyce M. Gilmour

Editing TLC: www.editingtlc.com

Cover & book layout designed by Craig Komins

Kömins Group: www.komins.com

Cover Photo: akg-images / Rabatti - Domingie

Only The Wounded May Serve / First edition
ISBN 978-0-692-79123-3 (pbk)

1. Self Help —Conduct of life. 2. Health & Wellness —Recovery & addiction. 3. Mental Health —Happiness. 3. Religion & Spirituality —Inspirational.
I. Title.

ISBN 978-0-692-79124-0 (ebook)

ONLY THE WOUNDED MAY SERVE
By Leo F. Armbrust

CONTENTS

Acknowledgments   10

Chapter One   **Why?**   11

Chapter Two   **The Pain and Suffering of Being Human**   15

Chapter Three   **Fear Leads to Suffering**   21

Chapter Four   **Seeing Who Is Within**   27

Chapter Five   **Our Greatest Obstacle**   32

Chapter Six   **Changing What We Can Control**   36

Chapter Seven   **Letting Go of What Controls Us**   43

Chapter Eight   **The Power We Possess**   47

Chapter Nine   **Where the Power Originates**   55

Chapter Ten   **Naked and Vulnerable**   58

Chapter Eleven   **The Pursuit of Happiness?**   61

Chapter Twelve   **Why We Choose to Do Good**   65

Chapter Thirteen   **Faith and Trust**   69

Chapter Fourteen   **Embracing One's Self**   72

Chapter Fifteen   **Our Source of Strength and Purpose**   75

Chapter Sixteen   **We Are Sources of Goodness**   81

Chapter Seventeen   **The Power to Make a Difference**   88

Chapter Eighteen   **The Consequences of Our Compassion**   91

Chapter Nineteen   **Our Priorities Help Define Us**   94

Chapter Twenty   **Controlling Our Concept of God**   97

Chapter Twenty-One   **When Religion Seeks to Control**   105

Chapter Twenty-Two   **What All Religions Can Teach Us**   118

Epilogue   121

About the Author: Leo F. Armbrust   125

Acknowledgments

It has been said that life is best lived looking forward, best understood, looking backward. As I look back over these past sixty-five years, I am blessed to have been surrounded by family, relatives, and friends who not only have enriched my life but also have helped me discover myself. Their presence has been a means, much like a lens, to allow me to see myself for who I truly am. They have also been mirrors reflecting back to me what at times I did not see.

I am grateful to those of you who have previewed this book, for your comments and contributions. To Craig Komins, my publisher, and to Joyce Gilmour, my editor, your dedication and hard work have made this book possible, a dream I have longed to make a reality. Thank you!

Thank you, one and all, parents, siblings, men and women from all walks of life and from all forms of friendship, your story, as well as mine hopefully is captured within these pages.

Chapter One

Why?

"Once upon a time..."

Shouldn't all stories have a warm and familiar beginning?

Well, "once upon a time" there was a man who wished to sail around the world. Some might say he wanted to circumnavigate the globe; of course, that's what they would say. He spent three years building a sailboat in which he sought to do so. After completing his work, he set sail from a port in California. Within a month, he had reached the southwestern Pacific. Unfortunately, a severe storm arose, the waves of which tossed his boat upon a coral reef and damaged his craft beyond repair. He swam to a nearby island and over the course of the next few weeks, he salvaged what he could from his wrecked boat. Over time, he resigned himself to the reality that he was marooned on a deserted island. What supplies he could rescue from the boat enabled him to construct a shelter against the elements. One day while scavenging for food on his island, he looked back toward the horizon to see smoke billowing in the sky. Quickly, he hurried back to his shelter only to discover it was being consumed by fire. Somehow, the embers from his campfire had caught his hut afire and had destroyed everything. All of his resources, his tools and supplies, were hopelessly lost. He screamed to the heavens, raising his fists he cursed God.

His bitterness and resentment welled up within him. After hours of complaining and crying in despair, he collapsed on the seashore. The next day he awoke to the waves on the incoming tide lapping against his face. As he raised himself from the sand, he was shocked to see a huge three-masted schooner at anchor in the lagoon, from which a small rowboat with two men in it approached the beach. At once, he leapt to his feet. Running into the water, he shouted to his rescuers, "How did you know I was here?" To which the men in the boat shot back, "We saw your signal fire!"

How many times in each of our lives has something happened which nearly broke us, emotionally, spiritually, mentally, socially, and/or even physically? At these moments in our lives we have struggled to go on, maybe we despaired, maybe we decided another course of action or chose another path for our lives. Whatever may have happened, this much is clear. A certainty we are oftentimes reluctant to admit: "Everything happens for a reason!"

Consider for a brief moment how different your life is now because of such tragedy or disaster that severely altered your life. Maybe you are still struggling with the "*why.*"

The great German poet, Rainer Marie Rilke, once wrote: "Be patient toward all that is unsolved in your heart and try to love the questions themselves, like locked rooms and like books that are now written in a foreign tongue. Do not seek the answers, which cannot be given you because you would not be able to live them. And the point is, to live everything. Live the questions now. Perhaps you will then gradually, without noticing it, live along some distant day into the answer."

Living with unanswered questions is one of the most difficult and challenging aspects of our lives. Why did he or she die? Why did I lose my job? Why did he or she leave me? What did I do to deserve this? Why did this happen to me? Why? Why? Why?

Yes, we are all too aware of others like ourselves who have suffered in a similar fashion. They too have no answers for some of their questions. Those whose opinion and counsel we seek and admire, are themselves without an answer. Like Rilke's insight, if we did discover the answer, we may not accept it, but resist it and eventually live in resentment because of it. The fact is this: many of the answers we could be given do not satisfy our quest to know the *why*. Just the offer of comfort in the phrase, "everything happens for a reason" does not appease us nor offer us solace for our deeply wounded self. We are left empty and frustrated.

Living with questions that go unanswered forces us to accept and live with mystery. Yet, we continuously yearn for the facts. We want the truth; living with uncertainty is far too much of a task for most of us. We prefer black and white more than gray. To place our faith and trust in what cannot be proven or defined is a leap far too many of us cannot make. The risk is surrender. Yes, surrender to a power we cannot understand let alone control. The very comment, "everything happens for a reason" posits a belief in a Higher Power, a power that is in control, which supposedly has our best interests at heart. That, in and of itself, is a stretch for us to acknowledge. We struggle to let go of what we consider our best interests to be. Who, after all, knows better than us what is best for us?

There may come a time when we ask ourselves, "Why should I even believe in a Higher Power?" No one can ever answer that question for you. It will always remain an answer you must discover for yourself. No one answer fits all of us. Neither the fear of punishment nor the desire for reward are sufficient enough to motivate each and every one of us. Many of us require a far more compelling reason, one that is profoundly personal, one that expresses a relationship of unconditional love. It is here that we come to a critical dimension whether we can move on from tragedy and disaster or remain fixed in a period of our lives that brought us to our knees or broke our hearts. Each of us knows someone who has never moved on; they willingly have elected to stay where they are, frozen in a time of suffering.

Whatever this event may have been, no matter the significance or degree of the pain and questioning, they are stuck. A similar metaphor is as one who drags an anchor. Each day he or she forges a new link of bitterness and resentment, as the length of chain increases over time, so too the effort to move even an inch becomes all the more impossible. Unless one opts to break the chain, their life will remain on hold; they are dying instead of living.

Moving on from our own unanswered questions is a life-changing decision. This transition from one place to another is more than merely physical; it is an emotional and spiritual step into a level of consciousness we did not know we possessed. It is a real journey into faith, for it demands self-surrender. It is a path where fear begins to diminish and is replaced by something far more powerful; the faith and trust that there is *always* a reason and answer, even if it remains unknown. Like all things vital and essential for life, we will never believe this until we undertake the journey and experience its potential.

Chapter Two

The Pain and Suffering of Being Human

My cousin is a farrier; most of us would call him a blacksmith. The Latin word for iron is "ferrum," hence the term. I have watched many like him ply their trade. They take a piece of metal and immerse it into an intense heat source. Slowly the metal becomes more pliable allowing the farrier to shape the shoes for the hooves of the horse. Retrieving the metal from the blazing fire, he takes the soon-to-be shoe and starts to pound it upon an anvil. The metal grows cold; consequently, he replaces it within the fire. This process continues until the shoes fit each individual hoof, for no two hooves are alike. The work is long and tedious, backbreaking and exhaustive. It is a craft that few have mastered and yet is so necessary for the horse.

The comparison is not too dissimilar from our own situations. We are shaped by both the emotional heat and coldness of our lives. We are molded and forged by events that pound us, weigh us down, and influence us. Just when we think our process of formation is complete, something or someone comes along and walks on us.

As humorous as this anecdote might seem, the reality is that we sometimes feel as though this happens to us. We have been deeply shaped and influenced by the struggles and challenges of our lives. Humanity has attempted to seek an answer to the question regarding the value of suffering in life. What is its meaning and purpose? What can be gained from such? If there is a Higher Power, why is this necessary? Are there no other means or methods to teach and form us?

The greatest fear we might have is this: that all of our pain and suffering might have no value. We are merely victims and we have nothing to gain from our unfortunate experiences. For any who engage in physical exercise, he or she is all too familiar with the expression, "no pain, no gain." Those who know the effort involved in such activity, know that physical exercise will eventually expand our muscles, our heart most importantly, to function on a better and higher capacity.

In a recent article from the *Wall Street Journal*, Daniel Cunitz writes about physical exercise/pain and indicates: "We don't do it because it is fun or in any sense pleasant; we do it because it is instructive. Nor does this apex level of hurt produce physical changes that make you more fit, it also produces mental adaptations that are ultimately more important. You learn that your perceived pain threshold is an illusion, that you are stronger, mentally and physically, than you had believed and that the normal discomforts of exercise, not to mention of quotidian existence, are laughable by comparison."

It stands to reason, as many propose, that human suffering has its own inherent purpose and meaning. None of us would be who we are unless we experienced some amount of pain and disappointment.

In *Man's Search for Meaning*, Viktor Frankl writes, "Life is a quest for meaning. The greatest task for any person is to find meaning in his or her life. Frankl saw three possible sources for meaning: in work (doing something significant), in love (caring for another person), and in courage (during difficult times)...

Suffering in and of itself is meaningless; we give our suffering meaning by the way in which we respond to it."

"I do not believe that sheer suffering teaches. If suffering alone taught, all the world would be wise. To suffering must be added mourning, understanding, patience, love, openness and the willingness to remain vulnerable." —Anne Morrow Lindbergh.

Pain is the price we pay for being alive. It does not come from God, only the strength to transcend it does. Expecting the world to treat you fairly because you are a religious person is like expecting the bull not to charge you because you are a vegetarian.

In *When Bad Things Happen to Good People*, Harold Kushner writes, "Laws of nature treat everyone alike. They do not make exceptions for good people or for useful people."

God is not in the flood or the earthquake, but rather in the people coming to gather to fix the damage. There will always be pockets of chaos and suffering in the world. Asking God to intervene or interfere would bring perfection but no goodness. Thus unquestioningly accepting the inevitably of pain is also the wrong answer. We must accept and embrace the facts that we as human beings, are often the cause for much of the pain and suffering, including our own, either by omission or commission. Likewise, we also bear responsibility for its remedy and repair.

In *When Bad Things Happen to Good People,* Harold Kushner writes, "God's pattern of reward and punishment seems arbitrary and without design, like the upside of a tapestry. But looked at from outside this life, from God's vantage point, every twist and knot is seen to have its place in a great design that adds up to a work of art... Belief in a world to come where the innocent are compensated for their suffering can help people endure the unfairness of life in this world without losing faith. But it can also be an excuse for not being troubled or outraged by injustice around us, and not using our God-given intelligence to try to do something about it... All we can do is try to rise beyond the question: 'Why did it happen?' And begin to ask the question, 'What do I do now that it has happened?'"

It can also be said that we have learned far more from failure than we have from success. Every failure we've experienced has taught us how much more is needed from us in order to succeed, to win, or to overcome. Failure can be the most valuable teacher we have if we allow it to become so, rather than wallow in the misery of our loss or shame. Regrettably, some cannot move on; they cannot accept defeat and learn from it.

Sometimes I ask people if they agree that failure has taught them more than success. Nearly 100% of the time they will assent that it did. Then I ask them, if it is true that failure is one of the most influential teachers in life, why would we ever deprive those we love from this necessary experience? Most will automatically state they do not want their loved ones to suffer, and yes, that is true. However, we cannot shield or prevent our loved ones from experiencing the failures, disappointments, and suffering of life, no matter how much we might try. The human condition is fraught with trials, loss, deprivation, weakness, and brokenness. Our greatest teachers have been failure and loss.

We may wrestle with the values of suffering, defeat, and disappointment, an ongoing human experience that has existed from the beginning of time and will no doubt persist as long as humanity survives. The lessons learned from failure or suffering are always conditioned by the ability of the one who suffers to comprehend their potential meaning. He or she must inevitably discover what it all means, even if the questions might never get answered.

In a recent article in the *Wall Street Journal* titled, "From Tibet, Sorely Needed Advice on Managing Pain," Melvin Konner writes, "Suffering is defeated through the end run of acceptance: You may have to keep the pain, but that doesn't mean you have to keep the suffering."

I once knew a married couple that had tried for more than five years to have children. Each time she became pregnant she would have another miscarriage. Both never lost hope. Sure enough, she gave birth to one of the most beautiful baby boys I have ever seen. However, in doing an initial examination of the infant, the doctors found a problem. With father in a medevac helicopter, in under an hour, both he and the newborn were transported to one of the best neo-natal hospitals in the state. Later that day, they both returned. The father took his son and placed him in his wife's arms. With tears streaming down his face, he told his wife that the doctors had discovered their son was born with half of a heart; there was nothing anyone could do to save the child. As I stood by both of them, the mother of this baby looked up at me and asked, "Can you tell me why God would ask to me to carry this baby in my womb for nine months and then take him from me?" I had no answer.

What would you say to her?

Any responses would be woefully inadequate to help or heal. Suggesting one now "has an angel in heaven" or "you can always adopt a child" trivializes the pain. Such well-intended comments are both seriously lacking in understanding and compassion. The fact is, there are no answers to give. There are only answers that both the mother and father must discover, if and when they choose to do so, or they must live with a question that might never be answered. In this particular case, it seems they did discover some answers, five of them to be exact. They adopted not one, not two, not three, not four, but five children. Yes, in the end, they had to live with a question and find answers the best way they could.

The need, or call it the willingness, to probe the questions of life are both normal and necessary. If we don't ask, we can never understand, nor will we ever know something, or someone. Maybe, in some, we can describe the resistance to ask the *why* as part of a much deeper issue, which would be fear. The fear of finding the real answer is more frightening than one might imagine. Tragically, in some cases, death will be their only form of healing. Ignorance and avoidance of the truth might seem better solutions. Either we ask, or we don't; if no answer is found, then we must choose whether we begin to live again or begin to die. There are no simple solutions, no easy answers, nor quick fixes. Expecting to suddenly see the light when one is clouded in doubt and darkness is unrealistic. Understanding and insight, like any substantial forms of healing are gradual, not immediate.

Chapter Three

Fear Leads to Suffering

In his book "The Alchemist," Paul Coelho writes: "The fear of suffering is worse than the suffering itself."

I know a person whose fear of visiting his dentist is so overwhelming that for weeks prior to the appointment he will have anxiety attacks sufficient to cause him heartburn and loss of sleep. While driving in his car to or waiting in the dental office, he will begin to sweat profusely. His clothes will be drenched in a bath of fear-fueled perspiration. When his visit is completed, the ordeal, as he often admits, will have been far less traumatic than his much feared anticipation and dread.

This is not uncommon, for we all know those who refuse to see their doctor simply because they are fearful of hearing bad news. Reflect on your own life for a brief moment. What fears have paralyzed you? What fears have prevented you from doing what is essential for your own happiness and peace of mind?

At first our fears are not so obvious; they reside well hidden, carefully disguised under an array of emotions that seek to cloak them. When we cannot control the people, events, or situations around us we become fearful.

Vice versa, fear demonstrates itself most readily when we are unable to exercise our control. The loss or absence of any control gives birth to a wide variety of fears. The corollary is all too true; fear creates a powerful need within us to control people and things around us. Whenever I have seen the all too popular bumper sticker that reads "God is my copilot," I want to shout to the driver of the automobile, "You need to change seats." Giving up control is never easy. Allowing ourselves to trust, even to trust God can be charged with fear.

Surrender is the opposite behavior of being fearful. Giving up such control enables one to confront and own one's fears, and ironically allows one to control them. The reverse is debilitating and self-destructive; when fears own us, they will control us, dominate us, and slowly erode our wellbeing.

One instance in daily life wherein most people manifest some fear is in air travel. The passengers are all too aware they have absolutely no control over their flight safety. They have surrendered their control to those in the flight cabin and the air traffic control towers. A surgical patient who will undergo anesthesia also faces a similar fearful situation; they are giving up control over their mind and body. The fear of never regaining consciousness confronts any person destined for surgery; for this reason some never elect surgery. Otherwise, they would have to confront the ultimate anxiety: death.

For anyone who has ever had the opportunity to take the adventurous ride called Space Mountain at Walt Disney World, then you are all too aware of what fear can do. For those who have never taken this terror-inducing trip, be aware of this: it is a roller coaster enveloped in total darkness, and I emphasize, *total* darkness. The passengers on this little excursion of utter dread and anxious intensity have no clue what awaits them: the unexpected dips and climbs, the sudden jolts to one's left or right, all produce screams heard throughout the enclosed structure. All the passengers can do is *react*; they have no other response. Most other roller coasters have clear paths that are obvious to the naked eye. I have often wondered, which is more fearful? That which we can see and anticipate or the fears we know exist and await us but have not yet manifested themselves? Much like life, when we have no control over the unforeseen turns and shifts of life, all most of us can do is scream. That's certainly one reaction.

As Yoda, the Jedi master would tell us: "Fear is the path to the dark side. Fear leads to anger. Anger leads to hate. Hate leads to suffering."

Fear is always the emotion that precedes anger. You probably don't believe that, do you? Well, consider this: someone shoves you in line at the supermarket, cuts you off in traffic, is rude to you on the telephone, or maybe someone is ignoring you or another is unresponsive to your requests. Each of these instances can be perceived as a threat to your self-respect and dignity. Feeling unimportant or undervalued increases one's fear of insignificance. No one, absolutely no one, wants to be regarded as worthless or without meaning, hence any sense of being treated in such an inferior manner raises one's fears. Anger is a consequence of such fear.

Be aware of this: no one can make you feel a certain emotion, no matter how much he or she might try. You are in charge of your feelings; when you lose control of yourself, others have gained control of you. Sometimes there are situations in which others may attempt to frighten you, threaten you, or instill even more fear in you. What is your response? Anger and retaliation seem the customary responses but what happens when you control your emotions and do not permit fear to control you?

In his book, *Man's Search for Meaning*, Frankl writes, "Forces beyond your control can take away everything you possess except one thing, your freedom to choose how you will respond to the situation. You cannot control what happens to you in life, but you can always control what you feel and do about what happens to you."

Fear gives birth to panic and panic restricts one's ability to breathe adequately; lack of oxygen inhibits one's ability to think clearly. Most people who panic in water, drown because of their inability to breathe properly. That seems obvious, doesn't it? Did you know every certified scuba diver is instructed *never* to stop breathing under water? In fact, divers are taught to regurgitate into their mouthpieces if the need arises to do so.

In *The Power of Full Engagement,* Jim Loehr writes, "The breath is a powerful tool for self-regulation — a means both to summon energy and to relax deeply. Extending the exhalation, for example, prompts a powerful wave of recovery. Breathing... lowers arousal and quiets not just the body but also the mind and the emotions. Deep, smooth, and rhythmic breathing is simultaneously a source of energy, alertness, and focus as well as relaxation, stillness, and quiet — the ultimate healthy pulse."

Remaining calm and breathing normally allows one to make better decisions in crisis situations. In the exact same manner, if we approach confrontations in life with the same behavior, we will make better decisions about what we say and how we react. Flying off the handle or losing our cool only exacerbates the problem. We have allowed our deepest fears to surface under the guise of anger.

I want to address another aspect of our feelings or emotions. That is, our feelings and emotions have absolutely no moral character. Let me repeat that; feelings and emotions have no morality. Only our actions, and our behavior have moral consequences. Feelings are both subjective and fickle; what we might feel today is easily changed tomorrow.

Eckhart Toll writes: "An emotion usually represents an amplified and energized thought pattern, and because of its often empowering energetic charge, it is not easy initially to stay present enough to be able to watch it... it wants to take you over, and it usually succeeds, unless there is enough presence within you."

Fear is such an emotion, so too is anger; neither has a moral quality but what they may motivate us to do very well has a moral quality to it. Thus, when someone asks you, "How can you feel this way?" they challenge or deny your feelings, which in effect, challenging or denying who and what you are. No doubt you will feel such rejection. Unless you're under control of your fears you only become all the more angry and upset. The fear of having one's feelings ignored or dismissed so casually increases one's fears of insignificance.

Remember your last argument with someone, how difficult it was to express your thoughts as well as your feelings. People can dismiss our opinions and disagree with our ideas but when one disregards our feelings and emotions, we take it far more personally. If you attempted to convey what you were feeling and the other person disputed or rebuked your feelings, then you felt it. You felt they disputed and rebuked the person you are, no doubt you took it very personally. Most disagreements between people occur and continue to last because they do not recognize the importance of understanding what the "other" is feeling. When anyone makes an effort to understand, "stand under" who we are and what we feel, then there is little question we have met someone who knows how to listen, not simply with his or her ears, but on a much deeper level, with their heart.

This is why it is so crucial for us to stop, listen, and observe another who is clearly angry and upset. Ask yourself, "Why is he or she so afraid?" Fear always precedes anger. Posing the question,

"Why are you afraid?" directly to the person who is displaying such anger may cause them to refute the premise, "I'm not afraid!" Again, many of us are reluctant to confront or even admit our fears, for it is an admission of weakness and vulnerability. Confessing such an Achilles' heel would only invite the potentiality of further control by someone over our fears. Only the truly strong and emotionally developed could allow that to happen. This however, is exactly what is so necessary and essential for any relationship of substance. Unless we do become vulnerable and open ourselves to someone we love, we will never be who we truly are; the other will attempt to love what is only a pretense.

In *Staring at the Sun*, Irvin Yalom writes, "You can't connect... unless you're willing to face your own equivalent fears and join with the other on common ground. To make that sacrifice for the other is the essence of a truly compassionate, empathic act. This willingness to experience one's own pain in concert with another has been a part of the healing traditions, both secular and religious, for centuries."

Chapter Four

Seeing Who Is Within

Years ago, I had the tremendous privilege of meeting one of the most beautiful actresses in the world. At the time, she was married to a professional athlete. In the course of our conversation, she became increasingly trusting of me. She told me something she later admitted on a well-known television program: "I never thought of myself as an attractive woman."

I was stunned by her candor and her failure to see herself as others did. Surely, no one would ever deny her physical beauty, yet she could not see it. Eventually, I came to this conclusion after this episode and others like it: "Others see in us what we do not see in ourselves."

Our own histories are replete with instances wherein someone saw in us what we did not recognize we possessed. Through their insight, patience, and persistence they helped us see what we could not.

The night was January 30, 1993; the location was the Beverly Hills Hotel in Beverly Hills, California. Standing in the front of the room that night before their biggest game of the year, was the head coach of the Dallas Cowboys, Jimmy Johnson. In front of him sat the 1992 Cowboy team. Jimmy addressed them in his usual manner; his voice reached a crescendo as he continued repeatedly to emphasize his theme: "The Buffalo Bills will turn the ball over," and "they will commit turnovers," and finally, "I can promise you they will make mistakes." Whether Jimmy was a seer and had access to a crystal ball is unknown but he was absolutely correct. The Buffalo Bills committed nine turnovers the next day, the most by any one team in Super Bowl history. How did Jimmy know? Or better yet, did he really know beforehand or did he simply convince his team they could force that many turnovers? Either way, the XXVII Super Bowl belonged to the Dallas Cowboys.

One of Coach Johnson's favorite quotes is from Johann von Goethe: "If you treat an individual as he is, he will remain as he is. But if you treat him as if he were what he ought to be and could be, he will become what he ought to be and could be."

How does one help another to discover such talent and skills that lie undiscovered and under-used? Consider this, in the words of William Arthur Ward: "The mediocre teacher tells. The good teacher explains. The superior teacher demonstrates. The great teacher inspires."

The great word "inspire" comes from the Latin "inspirare" which means to breathe life into, to animate, to excite and inflame.

The great artist Michelangelo Buonarroti once described sculpture as releasing figures imprisoned in stone. He had the unique ability of looking at a block of marble and seeing the figure trapped within. What a brilliant gift. Imagine teachers, coaches, managers, leaders, any person entrusted with the responsibility of guiding others, and how dramatically he or she might be in the lives of those in their care. For example, the word "education" comes from the Latin "e" (from) and "ducare" (to lead). Translated, this essentially means to lead or to bring out. Thus education in its truest sense is *not* what we give others but rather, what can be drawn out of them, what we help them see, what is already there, to discover and realize about themselves.

The truth is already within them; the real teacher breathes life into them, animates their inherent gifts, and helps them to actualize who they are.

Karl Rahner, the renowned Jesuit theologian addressed the topic of religious formation when he wrote: "The theological problem today is to find the art of drawing religion out of man, not pumping it into him. The redemption has happened. The Holy Spirit is in man. The art is to help men become what they are."

Legend has it that when Michelangelo completed his statue of Moses, a marvelous sculpture that resides in the Church of St. Peter In Chains, in Rome, that he surveyed his work, took his hammer and hit the knee of this great masterpiece and said, "Speak!" This great work indeed appears so life-like.

Great artists breathe life into their work. Great teachers breathe life into and inspire others to discover their inherent gifts, talents, and skills. Such masters help others see their true selves. There is another adage: "Whenever you see a turtle on a fence post, you know it didn't get there by itself." So too, each of us is a product of someone else's sacrifices, hard work, and example. They saw in us what we could not see, they believed in us when we could not believe, they did for us what we could not do alone, they helped us become who we are. Just as the Creator breathed life into Adam and Eve, it was the "Ruah," the breath/Spirit of God, who creates life itself.

Ralph Waldo Emerson once wrote: "Our chief want in life is somebody who can make us do what we can."

St. Augustine offered a theological insight that he quoted from St. Athanasius: "God became man so that man might become God." What a marvelous thought for everyone, even those who are not Christian, we are in the process of being Divine, fulfilling the design of the Creator's when He made us in His image and likeness. Yet we face a daily struggle to recognize the inherent worth and value we possess. Not unlike the actress I mentioned earlier, we struggle to see ourselves as we are, regardless of what others may think or say to help us. Thus, it remains a tremendous task for any master to enable his or her pupil to discover what lies within.

Our self-image, what we believe ourselves to be and who we believe we are, is without question the most critical factor in determining our peace of mind and our happiness in life.

There is an old Hindu legend which states that at one time all human beings were gods. However, they treated their divinity with such disrespect that Brahma, the chief god, decided their divinity should be taken away and hidden where humans would never find it. The question was, where to hide it? Should he bury it deep within the earth? Should he sink it to the deepest depths of the ocean? Or should he place it on the highest mountain peak?

Brahma thought for a long time it seemed there was no place on land or sea that humanity could not eventually reach. Finally, he decided, "I will place their divinity deep within themselves; they will never look for it there!"

Thus the most precious and significant truth about humanity was buried within itself. Ever since then we have been searching for the lost secret of our divinity. What a difference our lives would be if we could recognize that image of the divine within ourselves, even more, what if we chose to recognize it in others? What a difference that would make.

Human history is filled with attempts to find the Divine, either on a mountaintop, a forest, or some remote region of the earth. If the Divine could not be found in these places, humans constructed temples and structures to house Divinity. Eventually, some religions have moved from confining God to a place of stone or wood and placing the Divine in others, flesh and blood. God cannot be localized in material objects but only within human subjects. If we wish to find God, then we must look into human history. As long as society values buildings and places more than people, we will be blind to the presence of God in others, then the deaths of others will pale in comparison to the loss of a structure. It is for this reason that the Crusades had and continue to have such a questionable moral value.

The Divine is already here, within us, as T. S. Eliot wrote: "The end of all our exploring will be to arrive where we started and know the place for the first time."

In the Old Testament, men are called "gods" (Psalm 82:6). Even Jesus quotes the verse in John 10:34, "Is it not written in your law, 'I have said you are gods'?" Clearly, Judaism, Hinduism, and Christianity support the concept of Divinity already existing within humanity.

Chapter Five

Our Greatest Obstacle

The most significant task we will ever undertake is to accept and embrace our true self, not what we pretend to be, not what others expect us to be, nor what we don't want to be. For the greatest obstacle to self-acceptance is fear. Let me reemphasize: *The greatest obstacle to self-acceptance is fear.*

The great Jewish philosopher and theologian, Martin Buber, was a man for whom religion was much more about experience than dogma. He often told the story of an aged pious man named Rabbi Susya who began to grow fearful of his impending death. When his friends criticized him about such fear they would say, "What, are you afraid you will be reproached because you weren't Moses?" To which the rabbi would answer, "No, that I was not Susya."

Fear paralyzes us. Fear causes us to manifest an image that is not who we really are. As we discover our flaws and defects, aspects of our personality that we dislike, we begin to find ways to distract or to disguise them. The fear of others recognizing our vulnerability and wounds is so great that we succumb to some of the worst examples of human behavior. How could we ever recognize the Divine within us when our sole concentration is our flaws and weaknesses? We are blind to our inner beauty and inherent value.

Nearly four hundred years ago in the city of Florence, Italy, a block of purest marble lay behind the city's cathedral gathering dust and suffering from the effects of exposure to the elements. Originally, this magnificent block of marble was quarried at a great expense. Unfortunately, the stone had been damaged in its quarrying and its shipping, resulting in a huge gouge in the middle of the column.

One sculptor, Duccio, thought he could carve something from the piece but sadly he only made the damage worse. Finally, he gave up his efforts and his failure became known as the Duccio column, a flawed symbol of frustration and failure.

A generation of artists would come and go, each one examining the column to attempt a design that would overcome the horrible flaw in the middle of this expensive piece of stone. The Board of Works for the city of Florence found few proposals that merited their approval. There was a brief time when some thought that the great Leonardo da Vinci might undertake the effort to create something from the block. However, even he could not devise a design that would utilize the whole column. Da Vinci declared to the Florentine Board of Works during a public session that sculpting marble was the work of common laborers and not the work of real artists.

Da Vinci's words did not sit well with one particular spectator. He was a mere twenty-five years old and had been dreaming for years of carving the Duccio stone. This young artist had been admiring the column since he was a teenage apprentice in Florence. Returning from Rome many years later, he was relieved to see the block of marble still resting on its side behind the church. Motivated by da Vinci's scorn, he made a model of his vision for this piece of marble, a model he had been pondering for years. For months, he tried to persuade the Board of Works to grant him the commission to sculpt this marble. He very much wanted to give a statue to the citizens of Florence that they could be rightfully proud of in their city. It took the artist another three years to release the beautiful figure he saw imprisoned inside the column. Who was the artist? His name was Michelangelo and the masterpiece he carved, is none other than "The David." Michelangelo could see the dramatic tension of a swiveling figure of twenty-five degrees within the damaged column. Today, it is known as the "contrapposto pose."

Our greatest teachers, mentors, coaches, and witnesses helped us not only to see our idiosyncrasies, weaknesses, and errors, but equally important, they helped us to own them. When our fear of self-exposure dominates us, we cripple our ability to be honest and sincere.

Here again, the topic of sculpture and marble appear. The word for *sincere* comes to us in two words from the Latin "sine" (without) and "cero" (wax). Which essentially means without wax. Perfect pieces of marble, those lacking cracks and crevices were referred to as being "sine cero." The defects and blemishes of the imperfect marble would be filled with wax to hide them. The sincere person is *not* an individual without imperfections, but rather one without the means and the desire to hide them.

In his book, *The Religious Man*, Huston Smith tells of a true story in which one's self-discovery leads to a newfound sense of self-worth.

He was a typical freshman in a small Midwestern college, when one morning the professor he most respected opened the class by saying, "Last night I read some of the most significant words I have ever come across, and I want to share them with you." As he proceeded to read, the boy's heart leapt to his throat as he recognized his own words from a paper he had submitted the previous week. As he relates the incident: "I don't remember another thing that happened during that hour. But I shall never forget my feelings when I was brought to my senses by the closing bell. It was noon, and October was never so beautiful. I was exultant. If anyone had asked me for anything, I would have given it gladly, for I wanted nothing. I ached only to give to a world that had given so much to me."

The point is clear: If a young man found himself changed to this extent by the interest a mere man had shown him, is it difficult to imagine the change that would come over us if we realized how loved we are by God? Once again, the question looks us in the eye: "Why should I believe that God loves me?" And once again, that question is a lifelong pursuit, one that necessitates a relationship. For it is only in relationships that we discover who we are, therein we find our redemption from our weaknesses and salvation from our despair.

In *The Gift of Therapy*, Irvin Yalom writes, "A great many of our patients have conflicts in the realm of intimacy, and obtain help in therapy sheerly through experiencing an intimate relationship with the therapist. Some fear intimacy because they believe there is something basically unacceptable about them, something repugnant and unforgiveable. Given this, the act of revealing oneself fully to another and still being accepted may be the major vehicle of therapeutic help."

Recall that special moment when someone you loved deeply, confessed his or her love for you. Our world changes when we realize and understand the value others see in us. Others become a mirror that reflects back to us our own self-worth, despite our flaws and deficiencies; they love us for who we are. Therein lies *all* the difference, for there is nothing in existence that is more redeeming than *love*, nothing more restorative, nothing more meaningful and nothing more essential to life itself.

Chapter Six

Changing What We Can Control

Shortly before the start of World War II, a young couple became engaged and made plans to be married within the coming year. December 7, 1941 changed all of that. Despite the wishes of both of their parents to postpone the wedding, the couple married before the young husband was ultimately drafted into military service.

He was assigned to basic training in Arizona. There he would prepare himself for combat in the North African campaign. His new wife followed him and found an inexpensive place to rent just so they could be near each other. Only rarely, if ever, did they get that opportunity. For the new bride, life in the desert was beyond her strength and comprehension. The local Native Americans avoided her and gave her no inkling of changing their ways. Many refused to speak English to her. The desert seemed lifeless, barren, and boring; the heat was unbearable, 100 degrees in the shade. Six weeks of her stay would pass; one day she wrote a letter to her parents expressing her regret that she had not heeded their advice and postponed the wedding. She was miserable and no amount of love from her husband, whom she seldom saw, could remedy her misery.

As her mother read her daughter's letter, she knew all too well this was not the time to say, "I told you so." Instead, her mother wrote back to her and in the letter expressed her understanding for her daughter's plight. She sought to comfort and support her and included this quote from Dale Carnegie: "Two men looked out from prison bars: one saw the mud, the other saw the stars."

Reading her mother's letter, the young bride admitted to herself that she really had made no attempt to explore the surroundings or the people around her. For all intents and purposes she had remained a stranger in a strange land. She decided to change that. The very next day she went to the local library and started to read some books about the Arizona desert, the Native Americans, and the fauna and flora inhabiting the region. She began her research and over the course of the next few weeks, she never tired of her efforts to educate herself. Eventually she made some overtures to befriend some of the resident Native Americans. At first, they were suspicious of her intentions, but in time, they recognized her sincerity and interest in their culture and customs. More than a few of the locals befriended her; they would lead her out into the desert to show their ancient ancestral sites, teaching her their language and the art of weaving. They taught her their language and tribal rituals. Her husband was inevitably sent overseas but she remained in Arizona. An entire new world had opened for her. Over the course of her life, she has written several books about this desert, the Native Americans who live there, and the various species of wildlife that do as well.

What changed?

Certainly not the desert; it remained as it was before and during her stay. The heat was the same, neither the land nor the climate changed. So too, the Native Americans retained their language, customs, and traditions, nothing changed about them either. Very simply, the truth is, she changed her *attitude*; the one element over which she had total control.

One of the most difficult and frightening tasks in life is to change. Some changes are voluntary; most of the rest in life are not. We choose them, either reluctantly or willfully, but all of us know that change is an essential feature of life. Those who cannot adapt and evolve will inevitably perish. Heraclitus, the famous Greek philosopher once said, "The only thing that is permanent is change itself." According to him, the only constant is change. John Henry Newman wrote, "To live is to change; to be perfect is to have changed often."

Yet why do we resist it so often and with such vigor? The principle reason is obvious: we are afraid of the unknown. Fear can prevent us from doing the right thing, the only thing, and the necessary thing. Most would rather confine themselves to the known and the familiar than to risk the safety and security of the unusual, unconventional, and the different. Change in the nature and quality of a special relationship, change of employment, change of residence, change in one's health, change in one's thinking; these are but a few of some of the most dramatic transitions that happen in all of our lives, ultimately, even the change from life to death. I have met few people who have no fear of death itself; for some, the fear is not the *when* but the *how* that troubles them mostly.

In *Staring at the Sun*, Irvin Yalom writes, "Of those people who permit themselves to encounter death authentically and to integrate its shadow into their core being... it is the synergy between ideas and intimate connection with other people that is most effective both in diminishing death anxiety and in harnessing the awakening experience to effect personal change... great importance to many who ponder or face death... the positive correlation between the fear of death and the sense of unlived life... in other words, the more unlived your life, the greater your death anxiety... the more you fail to experience your life fully, the more you will fear death."

Changing one's attitude is a continuous feature and important part of one's life. It is easy to form an attitude about others, individually, collectively, ethnically, racially, whatever, based solely upon observation, what one may hear through others, or read in the media. These sources of information are not always reliable nor are they credible, yet there are many who base their attitudes solely upon these forms of communication. We know the so-called "facts" can be easily distorted, exaggerated, and embellished, but still there are many who believe most of what they read, what they hear, and are totally convinced by what they see.

Thich Nhat Hanh in his book, *Being Peace*, recounts a story by the Buddha in which a father was told his infant son had been kidnapped and murdered by robbers. The father grieved the loss of his son for many years. One day, the son he thought was dead escaped his captors and appeared at the door of his father's house. He knocked on the door repeatedly, saying he was his son, but the father refused to believe him and would not permit him to enter.

Thich Nhat Hanh further states: "Sometime, somewhere you take something to be the truth. If you cling to it so much, when the truth comes in person and knocks on your door, you will not open it."

Our senses are definitely not that reliable, yet we develop attitudes that shape our speech, our behavior, and our thinking. Until some major episode occurs, some dramatic event that seeks to disrupt our lives, our attitudes remain fixed.

In the New Testament, there is a story of Jesus of Nazareth multiplying the loaves and the fishes (Matthew 14:13-21 and Luke 9:16). In the story there are five thousand men gathered, not including the women and children. When Jesus instructed His disciples to feed all of the people, they responded by saying they only had five loaves and two fish. So Jesus took what little they gave Him and distributed it to those around Him. The story concludes by stating that everyone was satisfied and there were twelve baskets of food left over.

There are countless numbers of people who have imagined a mountain of bread and fish materializing right there in the midst of everyone. Or a basket that never empties of its contents and simply replenishes itself each time some food is taken. All of this is a product of imagination and makes Jesus more or less a magician; in reality, a greater miracle occurred.

As an aside, I well remember Mother Teresa's comment: "The garbage cans of America could feed the world."

In the first century A.D., no one would ever leave the confines of one's home or land without taking food and drink for the journey, no matter how short or how long. One could not rely on the hospitality or generosity of others, nor were there any restaurants or resources to feed those that traveled. Even the wells were either privately owned by an individual or by a tribe of people. All that anyone had to consume was what he or she brought for the trip. Consider the normal reaction by those amongst the five thousand, looking around one could see that others had more, still others had less or even nothing at all. The fear of giving something to another that might be required or needed later causes some to be far less generous, the rationale being, "If I give you what I have, I might not have enough for me and my family later." Thus, the fear of potential want or scarcity inhibits their charity toward others in need.

What Jesus did was to set an example for all those gathered that day; He shared what little He had with others around Him. Such an act of goodness and charity led others to do the same. No one would have believed there was so much food available that not only could all be fed, but there would be twelve baskets left over.

His greatest miracle was not to multiply the loaves and the fishes but rather to change the hearts and attitudes of all those who were there, those that were fearful of sharing with those around them. That was the real miracle. Changing someone's *attitude* is indeed a miracle of incredible proportions. To convince others to give not from surplus but from want is seemingly beyond everyday logic.

But isn't this exactly what we are called to do for others? How do we help others change their attitudes for the better? How do we motivate others to reach beyond their self-imposed limits? What can we do for others who persist in their ignorance and prejudice?

Asking anyone to ignore their fears and to leave their comfort zone is a monumental request. Unless one does seek to effect some change though, their lives will remain in a self-constructed prison of monotony and dormancy. For those who have borne the pain of a relative or friend suffering from alcohol or drug addiction, they are all too aware of the struggle to help their loved one change their lives for the better.

One of the well-known phrases in places of recovery is: "When the fear of remaining the same becomes greater than the fear of change, then we will change."

Yes, it may well take the dominance of one fear over another for us to embrace change in our lives. Rather than lose someone, our jobs, or our wellbeing, some people will accept change much more readily. The threat of losing something can be a strong motive for making such a decision.

Returning to the responsibility we have to ourselves and to others, we must examine our attitudes each and every day. Our fears have influenced nearly all of these dispositions; unfortunately, we do not detect such a force until it manifests itself. Spending some time in our day to be quiet, to be silent, and listen to our hearts is as important as any other activity for the benefit of our health, emotionally, spiritually, and physically. When we ignore the voice that speaks from within, we neglect the opportunity to understand and accept ourselves as we really are, not someone we imagine or pretend to be. To examine and know our attitudes is to explore our fears, to recognize our fears is to begin to uncover the true person within us.

Viktor Frankl put it very succinctly: "When we are no longer able to change a situation, we are challenged to change ourselves."

Chapter Seven

Letting Go of What Controls Us

One of my favorite books, one that I consistently pick up and read again and again is, *Love Is Letting Go Of Fear*, by Dr. Gerald Jampolsky. I highly recommend this book. In his book, Dr. Jampolsky writes: "Peace of mind as our single goal is the most potent motivating force we can have. To have inner peace we need to be consistent in having peace of mind as our single goal."

You may wonder, even ask yourself, is that possible? Well, it is if you are willing to accept the fact that our minds can choose our reality. When we employ words or beliefs such as "can't" or "that is impossible," then we have imposed limits and boundaries on our abilities and potential. So often our past fears have dictated our unwillingness to be free of what holds and confines us. Freedom from the past fears begins with our need to forgive ourselves and others for past failures, disappointments, and suffering. The initial step toward inner peace is the spirit of forgiveness we must instill. Not temporarily, not casually, or even individually, but an attitude of forgiveness that restores, erases, and eradicates any previous sin, failure, pain, or heartbreak.

The process of forgiveness is a struggle to place our feelings in a secondary status to another's. Often our pride will not allow this without a lingering sense of resentment and bitterness. Again, we confront the dragons that seek to control us, the feelings of betrayal, insecurity, embarrassment, jealousy, et al.

It has been said that when you love someone, you can forgive him or her anything. Anything? Yes, anything, absolutely *anything*! For only those you love can break your heart. You will never know how much you love someone until they push your boundaries, your limits of forgiveness. Then and only then will you discover whether you have the capacity to do so or not. If you cannot forgive them, then you did not love them as much as you thought you did. You may need to ask a Higher Power for the courage and strength to do so.

The fear of being betrayed, of being used or abused, the fear of our loss of significance will cause many to refuse forgiveness to others. All too many times we have witnessed those who have consigned themselves to past instances of rejection, deceit, suffering, and violence, completely and totally opposed to forgiveness. For these, the sentence is life in a prison, self-imposed, self-created, and self-supported.

Letting go of the past, with all its regrets, is undeniably a major step in one's pursuit of inner peace. All too often there have been moments when we have felt such a deep sense of shame about ourselves.

There is a significant difference between guilt and shame: guilt is how we feel about what we do, which is known as behavior; shame is how we feel about who we are, all the features and characteristics of our identity. Most importantly, we need to recognize we can change our behavior but we cannot change who we are. I cannot emphasize this enough.

If we research the historical movements of groups who felt marginalized, oppressed, or segregated, we will discover their efforts, both violent and otherwise, to exert their pursuit of justice, acceptance, and rights in society. The shame they felt is removed by their own convictions and heroic efforts. They could no longer believe nor tolerate that they were inferior or unwanted; such shame was deeply personal and imbedded within them. They could no longer accept the attitude or behavior that relegated them to a lack of dignity or self-worth. Those who had the power, control, and responsibility over others did not always treat those "beneath them" with the respect and dignity they deserved. Hence, the shame became a process of internal indoctrination, a means whereby one was led to believe they were unlovable, unwanted, and worthless. Who wouldn't begin to develop a sense of shame about factors beyond their control?

Behavior is changeable. Race, gender, sexual orientation, physical and intellectual abilities, etc., are just some of the factors that help define who a person is; these identifying elements are not so transitory. The shame that has been induced by others upon the weaker, the minority, and the misunderstood, has proven to be a struggle in history that expresses humanity's efforts to remove the barriers of fear that exist. Until and unless those barriers of fear are taken down, the shame will persist and consequently so will the anger and the hatred.

When we speak of guilt, we must study the effects of such an emotion. Guilt can be both constructive and destructive; it can motivate one to improve behavior or it can confine one to a moment in one's past from which they choose not to escape. Somehow, someway, they cannot forgive themselves; their punishment for such guilt is self-sentenced. Such personal persecution does little to heal or help the offender or the one offended; instead, it only regurgitates the same offense over and over again. Nothing can be learned from repeating one's mistakes.

Such self-penalizing activity only further exacerbates the problem. If we are reluctant and unwilling to forgive ourselves, just imagine how difficult it must be to forgive others who have offended us.

Chapter Eight

The Power We Possess

The most famous example of forgiveness in Scripture is the story of the Prodigal Son. Regardless of whether one is a Christian or not, there are some important lessons to be learned from this parable. Let's look at Luke, chapter 15:11-32, the only Gospel where it appears:

11 Then he said, "There was a man who had two sons."

12 The younger one said to his father, "Father, let me have the share of the estate that will come to me." So the father divided the property between them.

13 A few days later, the younger son got together everything he had and left for a distant country where he squandered his money on a life of debauchery.

14 When he had spent it all, that country experienced a severe famine, and now he began to feel the pinch;

15 so he hired himself out to one of the local inhabitants who put him on his farm to feed the pigs.

16 And he would willingly have filled himself with the husks the pigs were eating but no one would let him have them.

17 Then he came to his senses and said, "How many of my father's hired men have all the food they want and more, and here am I dying of hunger!

18 I will leave this place and go to my father and say, 'Father, I have sinned against heaven and against you;

19 I no longer deserve to be called your son; treat me as one of your hired men.'"

20 So he left the place and went back to his father. While he was still a long way off, his father saw him and was moved with pity. He ran to the boy, clasped him in his arms and kissed him.

21 Then his son said, "Father, I have sinned against heaven and against you. I no longer deserve to be called your son."

22 But the father said to his servants, "Quick! Bring out the best robe and put it on him; put a ring on his finger and sandals on his feet.

23 Bring the calf we have been fattening, and kill it; we will celebrate by having a feast,

24 because this son of mine was dead and has come back to life; he was lost and is found." And they began to celebrate.

25 Now the elder son was out in the fields, and on his way back, as he drew near the house, he could hear music and dancing.

26 Calling one of the servants he asked what it was all about.

27 The servant told him, "Your brother has come, and your father has killed the calf we had been fattening because he has got him back safe and sound."

28 He was angry then and refused to go in, and his father came out and began to urge him to come in;

29 but he retorted to his father, "All these years I have slaved for you and never once disobeyed any orders of yours, yet you never offered me so much as a kid for me to celebrate with my friends.

30 But, for this son of yours, when he comes back after swallowing up your property — he and his loose women and you kill the calf we had been fattening."

31 The father said, "My son, you are with me always and all I have is yours.

32 But it was only right we should celebrate and rejoice, because your brother here was dead and has come to life; he was lost and is found."

First, one must recognize that the younger son had absolutely no right to request that his father give him his share of the estate/inheritance. In ancient times and even into the twentieth century in some cultures, the estate of many families passed to the eldest or firstborn son upon the death of the father or patriarch of the family. Clearly, the younger son asked his father for something that he was legally not entitled to receive but also suggests the following: first, that his father must be dead, and secondly, he took from his older brother what was rightfully his.

The story relates how the younger son wasted all of his funds and resources on "wild living," essentially implying the most immoral and nefarious lifestyle. This might mean gambling, securing prostitutes, and any other form of activity contrary to Jewish law. Soon thereafter, his situation became worse; the foreign land in which he lived experienced famine. In order to survive, he found a job feeding the pigs. For a Jew, this was as low as one could sink; furthermore, he fed himself with the pigs' food. Yes, he had sunk to the depths of despair.

Eventually, the parable says, "He came to his senses." Deep within himself he was certain he could return to his father and find help. So he made his way home. It might appear to some that the son begins to rehearse his speech to his father.

Some may question whether his contrition is pure and his motive sincere. After all, he was starving. To others, it may seem he wanted only a clean bed and a good meal. Yet, we cannot deny this reality; he believed in his father's love for him, enough to draw him home. Be honest, even God works within those who have less than the best motives.

Ask yourself this question: Do you think it was a mere coincidence the father saw his son that particular day "a long way off"? Do you really believe it was an accident that the father happened to see him by sheer coincidence? I would wager that every day the father would stare down that road, yearning and waiting, just waiting with the utmost patience and persistence to see the son he loved return, walking to him upon that road. It was no accident, nor coincidence the father saw him that glorious day. He ran to the son for whom he had waited for so long. You see, the father knew his son would come home. Filled with such compassion, he embraced his youngest son. This action on behalf of the father was far more than paternal pity; it was unconditional forgiveness.

As his son poured forth his heart, expressing his remorse and contrition for his actions, the son was even willing to deny his relationship with his father, saying, "I no longer deserve to be called your son." The father would hear none of this, instructing his servants to "put a robe on him... a ring on his finger, sandals on his feet, and to kill the fatted calf." The father clearly announced it was a time to celebrate. Let's take a further look at the symbols of *robe, ring, sandals,* and the *fatted calf.*

The "robe" symbolizes restoration. The prodigal son who stood there in rags, tattered and torn, was now to be clad in vesture that revealed his status. He was the son of his father again. The "ring" signified great affection and a position of authority. Among the rich it was a sign of wealth and dignity, so the son was no longer impoverished or without status. Not only were his clothes those of a beggar, but he was also without sandals. In ancient biblical times, only servants and slaves went barefoot. Thus, the father would clearly state for the third and final time, his youngest son was not to be treated as a servant or a slave but as a son with all entitlements and rights.

Lastly, slaughtering the "fatted calf" was a celebration reserved for only the most notable and highly esteemed guest. Such an act was an expression of the respect that the host had for his guests.

When the eldest son discovers his brother has returned and sees his father's magnanimous response of forgiveness, he displays his true self. He cannot accept his brother, going so far as to disown him with the comment, "this son of yours." The older son demonstrates an attitude and a behavior not uncommon in those who pride themselves on their legal and moral conduct. Their stellar performance in keeping the rules, the law, and obeying the system only turned their hearts and minds to stone. They had no sense of mercy or compassion for those who erred or committed sins. All they knew was their own adherence to what was required. Such a legalistic attitude prevented the older brother from embracing a brother who had been lost and now was found.

Obviously, fidelity to the law did not necessarily render one with a deep sense of understanding or tenderness for the sinner. Instead, the legalist demanded recognition and reward for simply doing what he was required to do. For those like him, their motive was not so pure. They follow the commandments but refuse to love generously. Like so many who want so desperately to keep the rules, they also crave attention for their obedience. They react bitterly when one who does not obey is given what he or she believes is theirs. They cannot rejoice in the good fortune of another, rather they resent it. Children who see their parents acting unfairly usually see life the same way: "You never allowed me to drive the car at sixteen," "You never gave me a new bicycle at Christmas," "You never let me stay out past eleven o'clock." Do these comments sound familiar? These self-perceived snubs from what some felt they deserved continues into adulthood, a lifelong display of cynicism, bitterness, and resentment for being treated unfairly.

The father's love and forgiveness are unconditional. There was no requirement on the part of the prodigal son to repent, to perform some type of penance or public apology. There was only the father's incomprehensible manifestation of mercy. His actions defy both reason and logic. Notice what transpired: the son received from his father, restoration, reconciliation, and renewal. The son who was lost was not only found but it was as if he had never left; he remained his father's son, but this time with a new beginning and a new life.

The fairy tale story of Humpty Dumpty imparts a valuable lesson to all of us. We have the capacity to help others put themselves back together again. We are the "king's men" who can put Humpty Dumpty back together when he falls. When we forgive others who have offended us, we can reconcile and restore them from their separation and brokenness, even when they do not recognize their own sins or offenses. We can put people back together who have been broken in marriage, in friendship, in a partnership, in a conversation or in a way of life. We have that ability and strength to do what seems impossible.

In his book, *That Man Is You*, Louis Evely recounts a story from the French playwright, Jean Anouilh regarding the Last Judgment:

"The good are densely clustered at the gate of heaven, eager to march in, sure of their reserved seats, keyed up and bursting with impatience. All at once, a rumor starts spreading: 'It seems He's going to forgive those others, too!' For a minute, everyone is dumbfounded. They look at one another in disbelief, gasping and sputtering, 'After all the trouble I went through! If only I'd known this... I just can't get over it!' Exasperated, they work themselves into a fury and start cursing God, and at that very instant, they're damned.

"That was the final judgment, you see. They judged themselves, excommunicated themselves. Love appeared and they refused to acknowledge it. 'We don't know this man. We don't approve of a heaven that's open to every Tom, Dick, and Harry. We spurn this God who lets everyone off. We can't love a God who loves so foolishly.'

"And because they didn't love, *Love*, they did not recognize Him."

Sadly, there are some who are quite smug about their virtuous behavior and are sure of their reservations in eternal life. But when the idea of unconditional forgiveness and love present themselves as God's mode of being, these very same people reject such a notion. These so-called elect bewail their carefully cultivated virtues and calculated acts of self-denial in life. Their so-called obedience is only a facade, they are imposters; their loyalty and intentions are not as pure as they seem. They emphasize the justice of God and consequently misunderstand who He really is. *He is love and mercy*!

One of my favorite quotes concerning the incomprehensibility of God's mercy comes from St. Isaac the Syrian, a seventh century bishop: "Mercy and justice in one soul is like a man who worships God and the idols in one house. Mercy is opposed to justice. Justice is the equality of the even scale, for it gives to each as he deserves, and when it makes recompense, it does not incline to one side or show respect of persons. Mercy, on the other hand, is a sorrow and pity stirred up by goodness, and it compassionately inclines a man in the direction of all; it does not requite a man who is deserving of evil, and to him who is deserving of good it gives a double portion. If, therefore, it is evident that mercy belongs to the portion of righteousness, then justice belongs to the portion of wickedness. As grass and fire cannot coexist in one place, so justice and mercy cannot abide in one soul. As a grain of sand cannot counterbalance a great quantity of gold, so in comparison God's use of justice cannot counterbalance His mercy." (I.51, p.379)

Chapter Nine

Where the Power Originates

Dr. Robert H. Schuller was an author and evangelist who founded the Crystal Cathedral in Southern California. He once wrote, "The classical error of historical Christianity is that we have never started with the value of the person. Rather, we have started from the 'unworthiness' of the sinner, and that starting point has set the stage for the glorification of the human shame in Christian theology."

What value we possess consists in being made in the image and likeness of the Creator. We are more valuable than we know.

Many years ago, a friend of mine named Jim, was celebrating a special anniversary, twenty-five years in ministry. Gathered at a banquet to honor him on that evening were family, relatives, and friends who had been his greatest sources of strength, support, and guidance. Throughout the course of the meal, many rose to praise and express their appreciation for this man's service in the name of God and his church. At last, the honoree rose to offer a few personal thoughts from his years of ministry. He began by saying, "I want to ask each of you a question." He paused for effect. "What do you believe God will ask you when you finally come face to face with Him at the end of time?" A few raised their hands. He called on his nephew. "Uncle Jim, I think God is going to ask me, did you keep my commandments?" The minister looked at his nephew and responded, "Billy, I once thought as you. I, too, thought God would want to know if I obeyed His laws, but I don't think He will pose that question."

Jim's cousin stood and offered this thought: "I think God is going to ask me, do you love me?" Jim nodded his head at his cousin, but then suggested, "No, I, too, once thought as you," he continued. "That is a very good question, however I think God has another question reserved for each of us." With no further suggestions the minister said, "I believe the question God will ask each of us is this: 'Do you believe that I love you'?"

There is no greater abyss in which to fall, than the depths of despair, into one that leads one to believe that he or she is unlovable, even by God. Nothing is more self-destructive than a depleted sense of self-worth. Such self-loathing is brought about by the fear of seeing and accepting the person one truly is. Almost as if one says, "If I can't love myself, neither can God!"

Whenever one begins a trip in an airplane, the flight attendants instruct the passengers that in the case of a loss of cabin pressure, oxygen masks will drop from the ceiling. Parents are told to place their masks on first and then on their children. Initially this seems quite backward until one realizes the adults must assume the responsibilities that children cannot. In effect, according to the individual, one cannot give what one does not have. The phrase in Latin is "Nemo dat quod non habet." Translation: "No one gives what he does not have." Imagine how difficult, if not impossible, it is to love another person if one does not believe him/herself to be lovable. How can one truly love another if he or she does not love him/herself? You just can't give what you don't have.

Throughout our lives we are called upon to care for, attend to, and improve the many aspects of our personalities. Whatever that may entail, we know deep down inside that any efforts to educate, expand, enhance, or develop our talents and abilities only furthers our wellbeing and sense of worth. It is not selfish of us to place our "oxygen masks" on first when others may need them as well. When we exercise our desire to become better human beings, others around us will benefit as well. The more human, the more loving, the better educated, the healthier we are physically and emotionally, then we will be better able to place "oxygen masks" on those within the inner circle of our life.

So too, the experiences of life that have impacted us the most can be best interpreted in our willingness to help others learn from what we have experienced. We can empower others to believe in themselves from our own insights of struggle with self-doubt and self-loathing. Nothing is more humbling than to learn the truth about one's self, yet that does not mean a sentence of hopelessness or gloom. We undergo a process of self-examination when we choose to allow our personal trials to become critical life lessons for others. Our journey is a means to tell a story, not everyone's story, just ours. But the endeavor to explain, enlighten, and enliven the meaning of another's toils in life for their own edification and understanding breathes life where there might have been only suffocation and even death.

Yes, we have the power to resuscitate those who are gasping for meaning and purpose in their lives. Many, if not most, are unaware of their decreasing lack of what gives them life. There have been numerous studies conducted in this country by those who work with terminally ill patients in the end stages of their lives. Most have shown that these men and women look back on their lives and regret the many things they wanted to do but never did. They also regret the time and effort they did not dedicate to the most important relationships in their lives.

Chapter Ten

Naked and Vulnerable

Recall the final scene in the movie, *Saving Private Ryan*. Standing at the grave of Captain John Miller, a now elderly former Private James Ryan stares at the grave of the officer who led the unit assigned to find him and bring him home safely. Suddenly, Ryan's wife who had been behind him with the others in the family comes to her husband's side and asks him if he was all right. With tears in his eyes, he looks at her and says, "Tell me I've lived a good life; tell me I'm a good man."

No one wants to leave this world without having contributed some labor that has made life better for others or touched the hearts and souls of the needy. We yearn to make and be a difference in this world. We strive to leave a legacy. Yet, this is impossible unless we see within ourselves the ability and courage to do so. We must love who and what we are, despite our flaws, weaknesses, and limitations. If we choose to remain confined by our idiosyncrasies and defects, then we'll never unlock the potential within us to find ourselves in this life.

For this reason, we must confront, acknowledge, and own the fear that prevents us from being naked, vulnerable, and exposed.

Some years ago a very good friend of mine and I traveled to an island in the Caribbean. The morning after we arrived, we went to the concierge at the hotel and asked about the best beach on the island. He informed us it was within walking distance of the hotel, so off we went. Upon reaching the beach, a sign was posted: "Clothing Optional Beach." Our curiosity got the best of us; we could not resist the temptation to see others in the altogether. We should have known better. Sure enough, those most willing to shed their clothes were also those least deserving and appealing to the critical eye. They were overweight, over-tanned, under-toned, and overaged. The moral of the experience became obvious: only those who had weathered the years of criticism, both from others and themselves, were most comfortable just "being their naked selves." In reality, they had nothing to hide. They cared less of what others might think or say of their figures, appearance, or lack thereof. I wondered later, *Why does it take us so long to be who we really are? Why do we place so much value on the esteem and opinions of others about who we are?*

Obviously, those walking and lounging on that clothing optional beach that day demonstrated they had nothing to hide and were utterly disinterested in the thoughts and opinions of onlookers. Imagine what our lives might be like if we did not place so much emphasis on what others thought of us. Simply put, they just didn't care.

I once walked into a restaurant in the Florida Keys and there posted in the entrance was a sign which read: "We Can't Tell You the Way to Success, But We Can Tell You the Way to Failure: Try to Please Everyone."

Consider how much time and energy we expend trying to make others like us, think well of us, or agree with us. Often we undertake such goals at the risk of compromising who and what we really are. Our desire to please others is often a self-betrayal. We compromise our true feelings, beliefs, and values in order to enlist the agreement and acceptance of others. Such disloyalty to our real self can be one of the most disgusting realizations we make about ourselves in the stillness and scrutiny of self-exploration. We know, we always do, when we have sold ourselves down the river. Our real selves have been disowned and hidden from view; we were not comfortable to say what we felt or believed. We refused to be "Me." Why? That's easy. For fear we would not be accepted or liked by others.

Standing up for one's values, beliefs, and convictions always takes tremendous self-confidence and courage to be true to one's self no matter what. Like those gathered on the clothing optional beach, we must be willing to risk the rejection and criticism of others who do not like what they see, hear, or feel. Unless we are willing to ignore the need to please others in life, because we believe we need their acceptance and affirmation, then we will doom ourselves to a life of failure and despondency. Finding genuine happiness will be only one of the many pursuits that will forever elude us.

Yes, we often make the enormous mistake of thinking that happiness is an end in itself, that one day we will find it. The irony of happiness is this: "It finds us."

Chapter Eleven

The Pursuit of Happiness?

Viktor Frankl, in his book, *Man's Search for Meaning,* says: "The pursuit of happiness is self-defeating. The more directly you seek a pleasure, the more it eludes you. Happiness is a by-product, a side-effect of a reason to be happy: a person to love, a cause to be committed to, a God to love..."

Any belief that the acquisition of material objects, places to live, jobs to have, or status achieved will ensure happiness is purely delusional. Our happiness is a by-product of the way in which we live; it comes to us in the quiet moments of self-discovery, when we realize that we have remained true to ourselves, that we have made our relationships with loved ones the primary goals of our lives. Then and only then will we acknowledge that our priorities have brought us more joy and happiness than we could have ever imagined.

A mother once wrote to her daughter a few lines as the latter was going through the trials and tribulations of her first year of college: "Happiness is not a goal to be sought, but the by-product of a certain quality of living. God did not promise us a happy life, but an abundant life. Abundance means sampling all there is, laughter and tears, excitement and loneliness, success and failure. Who are we to think we have the right to demand only happiness in the midst of a largely unhappy world? It is the richness, the depth, the contrasts that lend to life its real beauty. My prayer for you and me is that we will have the courage to experience life in all its fullness, and in the integrity of that courage we may find that elusive dream called happiness."

This profound sense of a life "well-lived" slowly dawns upon us, like an aha moment. Then we may be tempted to say to ourselves, "Why did it take me so long to discover this truth?" Not unlike those at the clothing optional beach, why did it take them so long to be comfortable in their own skin, regardless of how it looked? If we are patient with ourselves, we will learn much more about life. That is why it has been said, "The older we get, the more like ourselves we truly become."

The Danish philosopher, Soren Kierkegaard, once wrote, "There is only one sin ultimately, and that is the steadfast refusal to be true to one's own self."

Deciding to be one's true self is a lifelong endeavor. Choosing to be liked for who you really are is far more significant than being "loved" for who others mistakenly think you are. How many times in our lives have we made the goal of pleasing others our top priority?

No doubt one of the greatest temptations we face each day of our lives is to be true to our principles and values; any compromise for the sake of approval and acceptance is self-defeating. Standing firm on our convictions for the proper reasons is strong evidence of both our integrity and our character. We cannot betray our true self and be at peace.

I once read a column by Rex Huppke in which he wrote, "As human beings, we are at our best when we can be ourselves, when we live without fear of judgment or the pressures of putting on airs."

Living with such transparency and openness requires great personal courage. For most, it would be utter stupidity to place one's self in such a vulnerable state. Frankly, it seems absurd. It would be a risk that a majority of us would never imagine, let alone pursue.

An Episcopal priest who lived in Boston once wrote, "To keep clear of concealment, to keep clear of the need for concealment—I cannot say how more and more that seems to me to be the glory of life. It is an awful hour when the necessity of hiding anything comes. The whole of life is different after that. When there are questions to be feared and eyes to be avoided and subjects that must not be touched, then the bloom of life is gone. Put off that day as long as possible. Put it off forever if you can."

Creating an environment and a space for others, as well as for ourself to be who we really are, is the quintessential place to be fully alive, for there we can be home with no pretense, no facades, and no fiction. We can be comfortable in our own skin, naked and vulnerable to life itself; we can become our authentic self.

Have we encouraged and allowed others to be who they are and not who or what *we* want them to be? Have we surrounded ourselves with others who inspire us and permit us to be our true selves? Or do we avoid them? Unless we can find those that give us the freedom to be who we really are, we will never find happiness or peace. For we live in a world that at times wants to make everyone the same and for most. this is so much safer and simpler.

What kind of world would we live in if everyone thought the same, acted the same, and believed the same? Life is beautiful because of its diversity, contrasts, and contradictions. How could we ever appreciate music without silence? How would we ever know the value of love without the experience of hatred or indifference?

How could we appreciate the beauty of a sunny day unless we had weathered the clouds of a stormy day? How could one know anything unless one advanced from ignorance to knowledge? We all need these polar opposites in order to appreciate and understand the vagaries of life. This means we must seek the willingness to have a fulfilling life, one that has its contrasts and contradictions. An abundant life teaches us that the true meaning of life is contradictory: in order to get we must give, in order to live we must die, in order to believe we must doubt, in order to love we must hate, in order to gain we must surrender, in order to win we must lose. There is no understanding of what the other means or entails until we experience them both as opposites. When we do, we learn to appreciate and accept its opposite.

One who accepts that his or her life will be characterized by opposites and contradictions will ultimately have a fulfilling life. This is a life filled not just with the positive, but also equally important, the negative. There will be light and there will be darkness, times of sheer joy and others of utter sadness; there will be moments of insight and understanding, still others of doubt and confusion. True holiness consists of a life of wholeness.

Chapter Twelve

Why We Choose to Do Good

The great existentialist philosopher, Jean Paul Sartre, tells a story of when he was a boy wherein he was about to commit a harmless prank. All of a sudden, it occurred to him that God might be watching. Thus, he made a decision at that moment of his life to free himself of the burden of the belief that such a God existed. Later in life, Sartre admitted that were it not for his boyhood misunderstanding of God, both he and God would have gotten along quite nicely. What had happened was that God was being used, perhaps with the very best of intentions, but God was being used to keep the boy in line. The results of such misrepresentation are predictable. The thirteenth century Dominican Theologian, Meister Eckhart, wrote, "To use God is to kill Him." Using God as a means to frighten or control is the surest way to destroy the true image of God.

How can that be, you might ask. God's laws and rules have always been portrayed as an expression of how He wants us to live, and you would be correct with that assessment. However, employing the concept of a God who is anything but a God of *love* and *mercy* first, is a gross misunderstanding of God. The psychologist Lawrence Kolhberg helps to demonstrate this when he wrote of the six stages of moral development. The first level is that of Preconventional Morality, Stage 1, Obedience and Punishment (obeying the rules is important because it means a reward or an avoidance of punishment); Stage 2 is Individualism and Exchange (at this stage the individual chooses to evaluate the moral quality of one's actions based on whether or not one's interests or needs are met); second level is Conventional Morality, Stage 3 concerns Interpersonal Relationships (this stage reflects one's orientation to obey or comply based upon living up to the social expectations and roles of others); Stage 4, Maintaining Social Order (this stage is when individuals consider the good of society as a whole when making judgments, the focus becomes the maintenance of law and order by following the rules, doing one's duty, and respecting authority); and the third level, Postconventional Morality, Stage 5 (at this stage individuals start to account for differing values, opinions, beliefs of other people. The rules and laws are important for maintaining a civilized society, but the members must agree on these standards); Stage 6, Universal Principles (here Kolhberg's final stage of moral development is moral reasoning which is based upon universal ethical principles of justice, even if they conflict with laws and rules of society). This final stage reflects the highest form in the development and formation of one's conscience.

What stage do you believe the older son exhibited in his response to obeying his father in the story of the Prodigal Son? One can detect the movement from a self-centered purpose for being moral, to an other-centered one that places morality on a higher plane, the very essence and reason for morality, which is the highest good, *love* itself.

What does all of this mean? The highest motive for doing good and avoiding evil is based upon justice: what we owe to everyone, and why we owe it, because in the final analysis, we are called to love everyone. Hence, the highest motive for doing anything is the motive of love, not fear of punishment, nor desire for reward, nor is it the expectations of others or the pressure of conforming. We choose to do *good* because of what the *good* is. What is that *good*? It is what each of us comes to discover, what touches our innermost being, what appeals to our higher sense of reason and purpose. For most, this can be summed up in the simple phrase: "To truly live, is to love truly!" If there is a higher *good*, a more virtuous and fulfilling pursuit in life, it has yet to be found.

Herein we encounter another obstacle to developing our human potential: the motives and reasons for seeking and doing good in our lives. From Kohlberg's theory there are many who cannot evolve beyond certain stages; we've met and known them all. They cannot move beyond "reward and punishment," the "pressure to conform," the "need for law and order," etc. Very few progress to a level of doing *good*, because the norm is *love*. For most, it seems too naïve, too unrealistic for life. Such an approach appears to be ill equipped to face the problems and challenges of human interaction. Turning the other cheek only guarantees one a black eye and a wounded ego. Try doing that in today's world and one will most assuredly get run over or run out of business. It's kill or be killed.

This brings to mind the words of G. K. Chesterton regarding Christianity: "Christianity has not been tried and found wanting, it has been tried and found difficult." Not just Christianity, but any form of religious teaching that endorses not only the Spirit of Love but equally so, its practice in ordinary human behavior.

If we are truly willing to subscribe to the tenet that *love* is the absence of *fear*, then it only seems logical that we must let go of our fears in order to be more loving. In fact, the very issue is, we are far too suspicious, even fearful that such a commandment to love others is far too idealistic and can never really work in this world, maybe the next, but certainly not this one. Therein lies our dilemma. Is it any surprise then that we continue to suffer from many of our own self-imposed fears? Love is the total absence of fear. As Albert Einstein once wrote: "A man's ethical behavior should be based on sympathy, education, and social ties and needs; no religious basis is necessary. Man would indeed be in a poor way if he had to be restrained by fear of punishment and hope of reward after death."

Chapter Thirteen

Faith and Trust

Developmental psychologists believe we are all born with two fears; the others we acquire or develop throughout life. Those two fears are: fear of falling and fear of loud noises.

"Fear is useless, what is needed is trust!" Mark 5:36 and Luke 8:50.

Faith and *trust* have been substituted for each other quite often in this text. *Faith* implies an intellectual and to some degree, emotional assent to a person or body of beliefs. *Trust* is far more personal.

Bertrand Russell once defined *faith* in this manner: "We may define faith as a firm belief in something for which there is no evidence. When there is evidence, no one speaks of faith. We do not speak of faith that two and two are four or that earth is round. We only speak of faith when we wish to substitute emotion for evidence."

I once heard the story of a circus performer who consistently amazed his audiences by tightrope walking across a high wire without ever using the security of a safety net. Whenever and wherever he performed this death-defying act, crowds of people would watch in amazement at his courage. Each evening he walked from one end of the high wire to the other with the ease of someone walking on solid ground. On one particular evening, he paused at one end of the wire and shouted down to the anxious crowd, "How many of you have believe in me that I can do this again?" Without hesitation, everyone shouted they did. Sure enough, he did it again. Then he did something highly unusual; he lowered a rope and had one of his attendants attach it to a wheelbarrow. Whereupon the high wire walker pulled the wheelbarrow up to the platform on which he was standing. Once again, he looked down at the people below him and asked them, "How many of you believe that I can push this wheelbarrow across this wire?" Without hesitation, they all applauded. One man stood up and shouted, "I'm certain you can do it!" The tightrope walker looked down at the man and asked him, "Sir, do you trust me?" To which the man quickly replied, "Of course I do." The performer responded, "Well, then, come up here and get in the wheelbarrow!"

Trust, is far more personal; it is also spiritual. There is a far more psychological distance with faith; it is primarily academic in nature. We can lose our faith in someone, but when he or she violates our trust, then such a tragedy will be felt on many levels of our personhood. Trust conveys a deeper commitment to another, something a great deal more precious. Because of such value, our fear of trusting others becomes the greatest obstacle to love in a relationship. A couple cannot advance to a higher, more fulfilling relationship until one abandons his or her fears and becomes vulnerable to the other.

The following is written by Harry James Cargas: "When the male albatross courts the female, he makes obvious his intentions by raising one wing in such a manner that he makes himself vulnerable to attack. In effect, he is saying I trust you. My purposes are honorable and with this act of trust, I prove it. This creature presents a tremendous lesson for us in this act of faith. Are we willing to risk as much to prove our own love? Loving is a risk and we are all engaged to some degree in a community of risk.

"The degree to which we immerse ourselves in this community may well be the measure by which we can realize our wholeness as persons. In loving, we choose to make ourselves vulnerable; we say to another person that our relationship will not be based on fear. We will be honest with one another. You might learn things about me over which other people might laugh. I believe that you will not laugh, you will learn things about me which other people might become angry or disappointed. I bare my soul to you in a manner in which you can ravage it, if you choose; I trust that you will not ravage but love instead... We must be sensitive to others so when they lift their wings to us, we do not attack their weak spots. It is not easy to do so, but loving does not seek the easy route. Even when we feel we have been misunderstood or have been attacked, if we are sincere lovers, we will not attack in return. To love sometimes means to absorb pain. And if we make this an integral part of our own personal attitudes, we will not limit ourselves to one person or one family but extend our love as widely as we can."

Allowing one's self to be naked, exposed, and transparent is without question one of the most signature events of our lives. It marks the time when we refuse to be held back, when we deliberately choose to admit our fears and own them. They can no longer control us because of our unwillingness to identify them nor can they restrict us from the risk of vulnerability. This is a liberating moment; one that gives a greater sense of freedom and self-actualization.

Chapter Fourteen

Embracing One's Self

In 1935, two men, Bill Wilson (Bill W.) and Dr. Bob Smith (Dr. Bob), founded Alcoholics Anonymous in Akron, Ohio. The two men had gotten together, and being honest, admitted to each other that they were alcoholics. They realized the seriousness of their problem not only for themselves but for others, too. Both men decided they were going to make every effort to help other people recover from alcoholism. They started to work, individually and together.

Weeks and months went by, and after a year they found themselves sitting once again in the same office, they had been in where they made a decision and a commitment to help other alcoholics become sober. They seemed discouraged for neither one of them could truthfully say that he had actually helped anyone return to sobriety. Then the thought occurred to both of them: we are alcoholics and both of us have been sober for an entire year! By our efforts to help others, we have actually helped ourselves. That was the beginning of AA.

I believe one of the greatest spiritual courses ever devised are the Twelve Steps of Alcoholics Anonymous. In these twelve steps, one confronts the deeper realities of one's life. The movement from acceptance to ownership, to contrition, to making amends for their alcoholism is indeed a journey that is carefully constructed and purposefully orchestrated. The success of this transition demands openness and honesty. Whenever one attends an AA meeting, those present who are alcoholics

ONLY THE WOUNDED MAY SERVE

introduce themselves, giving their first names and adding, "And I'm an alcoholic." There is no pretense or attempt to hide one's identity; the alcoholic admits and accepts who he or she is.

Once again, we come to the difference between shame and guilt. Guilt concerns one's behavior or the lack thereof; shame concerns one's identity. Notice there is no shame in confessing one's self in this instance. However, the entire purpose for one's admission of such is to learn to control one's addiction. Every alcoholic in AA must admit that this disease is beyond his or her control and without the surrender to a Higher Power and the support of others, he or she cannot control this disease. Trust me, folks, that ain't easy by any stretch of one's imagination.

The greatest conquest we undertake in life is not "out there." No, in fact, it is within each of us; yes, it resides within us. On some occasions, we are more than ready to do battle against the forces within us that seek to undermine our strongest values and our most ardent beliefs. We are tempted to ignore or compromise what we have taken an entire lifetime to discover and learn. We are seduced by pressures to conform or simply abandon our very principles. The test is ongoing; it never seems to tire in its relentless effort to lure us into a false world, one that seems so real but in reality is both dark and miserable. Unless we have spent any time there, few if any of us will recognize its deceptions.

There can be no relief or joy in what is fleeting, insatiable, or lacking substance. Succumbing to the movements and pursuits of the herd may render our individuality and uniqueness absent and meaningless. Societally speaking, this is an epidemic. We must be ourselves, true to ourselves, as is often said, everyone else is already taken up.

Being different is risky. It makes us "stick out." Any venture to elevate ourselves above the crowd makes us easy targets. That's a big gamble.

The most frightening and threatening people in life are those who don't care what others think or say about them. The same can be said of those in battle. The most fearsome warrior is the one who is not afraid of death. He does not run from it, he confronts it; most of all, he accepts its possibility. Relinquishing the fears that capture us begins between our ears. That's where the battle resides. Our minds have shaped and influenced us enough that all too often they have not been our best ally but in actuality, betrayed us.

Chapter Fifteen

Our Source of Strength and Purpose

Before he died in 1890, the great artist Vincent Van Gogh produced over 1,700 paintings and drawings, yet he only sold one of them in his lifetime for a mere eighty-five dollars. Van Gogh died believing he was a failure as an artist. Today there are seven of his paintings that ranked in the top thirty as the most expensive paintings of all time, from a low of $47.5 million to $82.5 million. He never had the opportunity to see how much his art would be valued. Van Gogh's immense collection did not convince him that his art would ever be so highly regarded by art collectors and art critics alike, yet he never stopped painting or drawing. What drove him to such persistence and determination? Was he insecure, insane, physically ill, plagued by bouts of depression, or driven to excellence? We cannot know for certain. He died of a gunshot to his head and though no gun was ever found, it is thought that it was self-inflicted.

How sad and unfortunate that one of the greatest artists of all time could not exorcise himself from his own demons. Yet it was those same demons that may well have enabled him to paint with such great vision and style. There are times when our flaws and weaknesses enable us to achieve a greatness that we otherwise would never attain. What are our imperfections, defects, and shortcomings? How have we used them to create and to attain a deeper purpose for ourselves? What's our recipe for lemonade when life seems to hand us a basket of lemons?

As we noted earlier, each of us has known an instance in our lives that has proven to be a defining moment, one that changed us on every level from what we were one day until the next. More times than not, this moment was one that brought us heartbreak, suffering, and sorrow. How we responded to this has made all the difference in our lives. The incredible power to transform a life-changing event into something good eventually defines our character.

There was a story about a shoemaker in France. One day his young son was playing on the shop floor when suddenly the shoemaker's leather hole punch, known as an awl, accidently rolled off the workbench and punctured the right eye of the boy. Eventually, the boy would lose sight in both of his eyes because of this tragic accident. This boy could have grown up as an angry and bitter person because of his unfortunate injury. Instead, much to his credit, one day he would take the very same instrument that cost his eyesight and design an alphabetic system of reading and writing for the blind by making small indentations on paper. The boy's name was Louis Braille.

Truly, in our weaknesses, in our frailties, and in our deepest suffering, we have encountered an aspect of who we are that has given us an insight into ourselves, where we would otherwise have never encountered. In tragedy and humiliation, in loss and deprivation, in doubt and despair, we met a crisis; we go on or we stop and die. This was a moment when the hammer hit the anvil and we found ourselves between both.

In his play, "The Angel That Troubled the Waters," Thornton Wilder wrote about a physician who approaches the pool at Bethsaida in order to be healed. (Recall the story of this pool in the Gospel of John, chapter 5). He waits like so many others for the waters to be "troubled" so he might be healed and made whole again. The angel who stirs the waters of the pool appears to him and says, "Stand back. Healing is not for you. Without your wound, where would your power be? It is your very remorse that makes your low voice tremble into the hearts of men. We ourselves, the very angels of God in heaven, cannot persuade the wretched and blundering children of earth as can one human being broken on the wheels of living. In love's service, only the wounded soldiers can serve."

A physician need not have cancer in order to adequately attend to the medical needs of his or her oncology patients. Yet there is little question that anyone who has a defect, wound, scar, or hurtful experience can be much more sympathetic to those who have the same. In slang expressions for those who treat addicts, it is often said, "You can't bullshit a bullshitter!"

"The great illusion of leadership is to think that man can be led out of the desert by someone who has never been there." — Henri J.M. Nouwen, *The Wounded Healer: Ministry in Contemporary Society*.

I recall a biopsy I underwent some years ago. As I lay upon the examination table I experienced some of the most horrific pain I have ever felt. After the biopsy was completed I looked down to see a rather frightening pool of blood about my waist. I looked up at the physician, just less than ten years my junior and posed this question to him: "You've never had this procedure, have you?" By his initial reaction of looking away from me, I could already predict his answer. He said, "No." Later, as I met with my primary care physician, I told him of my experience. He confessed to me that the methods were indeed medieval, barbaric, and humbling to say the least. Thankfully, no cancer cells were found; however, the ordeal left me angry. Why? Because of my fear of ever being required to undergo this procedure again. In some respects, I felt forsaken by the physician; I did not believe he was completely honest with me or candid in what the procedure might entail. As I reflect on this experience, I find myself fearful, betrayed, and disrespected, all contributing to my anger and disappointment.

Maybe, just maybe, the sympathetic voice and protocol of one who had gone through the very same nightmare might have assuaged and tempered my pain and anxiety, maybe not. This much is certain: one who has known and felt an impending incident we might dread is more often than not the one whose insight and advice we seek the most. There is much to be said for "personal experience."

In life, those who have walked the walk, rather than simply talked the talk, have more credibility than the latter. It has been written, that experience is a great school, but its tuition is very high. When we analyze the experiences of our past, we can ascertain those that bring us a smile and those that bring us regret and those that come with tears. Each and every one of them, regardless of how difficult and painful it is to accept, has a value beyond price.

Through our own travails, struggles, and defeats, we can help others to accept and embrace their own; whenever we meet another overpowered by fear, we can hold their hand, offer a shoulder to lean on and an understanding heart; whatever way this may occur, we may encounter those that could benefit from our journey. We have the opportunity when we make ourselves available, when we choose to be open and honest about our own fears and trials. Nothing can happen on our behalf to help others unless we have the courage to let our wounds be evident. One must assuredly like the wounds as much as the medals and awards one receives in life. Society however, most often sees the latter far more significant than the former.

To harken back to AA, the success of this organization is based on its ability to help others with the same disease. It would never have attained the results and renown it has, had it not been founded on the conviction that people, other alcoholics, especially one's sponsor, have a common bond, unconditional acceptance, understanding, and tolerance.

It may be said, that those who strive to do good in this world, those who seek to make a difference for the betterment of all, truly manifest the Spirit of God, who is *love*. If any would aspire to this rank, he or she must know this, today and forever: "In the army of God, only the wounded may serve!" — Thornton Wilder. Embrace, accept, and rejoice in your wounds, above all, like yourself because of them! "If you have no wounds, how can you know you're alive?" — Edward Albee, *The Play about the Baby*.

I am reminded of the story of a Protestant minister in the early twentieth century who decried and criticized the thought of people flying, saying, "If God had wanted man to fly, He would have given him wings." His last name was Wright; fortunately, this man had two sons, Wilbur and Orville, who responded to their father's criticism with the statement, "God may not have given us the wings to fly, but He did give us the brains to learn how."

We have been endowed with the remarkable gifts of intelligence and free will. We have the power and wisdom to make a significant difference. We have the potential to influence so many other people. We possess the skills to lead and to enlighten. We have the gift of helping others see their potential. We have a role in this world's direction.

The great British theologian and writer, John Henry Cardinal Newman wrote this prayer: "God has committed some work to me which He has not committed to another. I have a mission, I may never know it in this life, but I shall be told it in the next. I shall do good... Therefore I will trust Him. Whatever and wherever I am, I can never be thrown away. If I am in sickness my sickness may serve Him; if I am in sorrow my sorrow may serve Him. God does nothing in vain, He may prolong my life, he may shorten it; He knows what He is about... O my God, I will put myself without reserve into your hands."

A missionary became lost in a remote region of Africa. He stumbled for hours in the dense jungle and became ever more lost by the minute. Finally, he found himself in a clearing. There in the middle of which was a small hut with an African man sitting in front of it. The missionary was able to communicate with the man, explained his situation, and then asked the man for assistance in leading him out of the jungle. The African agreed to help the missionary.

So they started their journey out and back to the missionary's village. The African led and the missionary followed. For more than an hour, they trudged through the unmarked jungle. The missionary grew worried and anxious. He asked the man, "Are you sure this is the way? Where is the path?" To which the African replied, "Bwana, in this place, I am the path!" We have the abilities and capacities to be the paths for others to take. We know the way, simply because we have gone that way. In so doing, we have become the way for others.

Chapter Sixteen

We Are Sources of Goodness

There is a legendary story about an Italian village in the eighteenth century that was celebrating the 1000th anniversary of its founding. The village was located in a section of Italy that was renowned for its Pinot Grigio, an Italian white wine known for its dry, crisp, and food-friendly flavor. The mayor and town council voted to host a weeklong celebration in honor of the anniversary. It would be a birthday party like no one had ever seen. There would be music, dancing, and food, lots of food and of course wine, more than anyone could imagine.

Furthermore, it was decided to invite the vintners of the region to contribute some of their best Pinot Grigio for the feast. The families which owned the vineyards had planted and cultivated these precious vines for centuries, each competing against the other for recognition of the finest wine for that year. The mayor and town elders decided to construct a huge wooden vat in the center of the village and invite each of the many winemakers to bring their barrels and pour them into the vat so that all might enjoy the very finest of the wines. Everyone agreed to participate. So all the winemaking families brought their wine and poured it into the vat that was situated in the town square. Proudly, the heads of each family stepped forward, lifted their barrels, and poured in their prized wine. Cheers and shouts erupted from the crowd, from people who had come from all over the region, and some traveling many miles to join the celebration.

After the last barrel was poured into the vat, it was the mayor's privileged task to draw the first glass. Slowly he stepped forward to this huge wooden cask, turned the wooden spigot and drew the first glass, filling it to the top. He lifted the glass and toasted the town. He proceeded to take a very generous swallow and suddenly an expression of total bewilderment came over his face. He took another drink and again an expression of disbelief appeared upon his face. He then passed the glass to members of the town council and they too looked confused and shocked.

Why the looks of confusion and amazement? That's simple. You see, the problem was this: there was no wine in the vat. It contained only water. Every one of the families who were asked to give their best gave only water. Each was afraid their very best effort or contribution would get lost amongst the rest, so instead of giving their best, they gave nothing at all.

Without question, we have been hesitant to contribute our finest gifts or our best offerings when the possibility exists that they may become lost or unnoticed. We enjoy and appreciate the recognition and respect of others when it comes to our efforts and sacrifices. Any blindness to our hard work or generosity can be interpreted as use or abuse. The fear of such leads some to withhold their best.

It has also been said that the true character of any person is revealed by the way he or she treats someone who can do absolutely nothing for him or her.

How important are we in the grand scheme of things for the betterment of this world and for the sake of humanity? How necessary are we in the mind of our Creator? Abraham Heschel wrote the following: "Man is not an innocent bystander in the cosmic drama. There is more kinship with the Divine than we are able to believe. The souls of men are candles of the Lord, lit on the cosmic way, rather than the fireworks produced by the combustion of nature's explosive compositions, and every soul is indispensable to Him."

We cannot stand idle when there is so much to do, so much to give when so many need what we alone might be able to offer or provide to those who are lost, in need, or simply worn down by the struggles of life.

Another story from the life of Jesus that reflects His need for our involvement and our contributions can be read in Luke's Gospel, chapter 5, seen below:

1 Now it happened that he was standing one day by the Lake of Gennesaret, with the crowd pressing round him listening to the word of God,

2 when he caught sight of two boats at the water's edge. The fishermen had gotten out of them and were washing their nets.

3 He got into one of the boats — it was Simon's — and asked him to put out a little from the shore. Then he sat down and taught the crowds from the boat.

4 When he had finished speaking, he said to Simon, "Put out into deep water and pay out your nets for a catch."

5 Simon replied, "Master, we worked hard all night long and caught nothing, but if you say so, I will pay out the nets."

6 And when they had done this, they netted such a huge number of fish that their nets began to tear,

7 so they signaled to their companions in the other boat to come and help them; when these came, they filled both boats to the point of sinking.

8 When Simon Peter saw this, he fell at the knees of Jesus saying, "Leave me, Lord; I am a sinful man."

9 For he and all his companions were completely awestruck at the catch they had made;

10 so also were James and John, sons of Zebedee, who were Simon's partners. But Jesus said to Simon, "Do not be afraid; from now on it is people you will be catching."

11 Then, bringing their boats back to land they left everything and followed him.

While the disciples were indeed profoundly moved by the tremendous catch of fish and thus chose to leave their boats and everything behind to follow Him, there is another more important lesson to be learned. Consider this for a moment: if Jesus truly wanted to do something awesome and convincing, then why not just stand on the seashore, whistle, and make the fish jump out of the water and onto the beach? That would most assuredly have made a lasting impression. Once again, He avoided the temptation to act as a magician. This type of magical power would ensure that following Him would mean they'd never be hungry. But this is not the point of the story. The emphasis is, Jesus needs us to help Him save others. He needs us to continue His work, hence the story concludes with Peter and the others choosing to leave their careers as fishermen and following Him. That is the point: they saw they were needed and they responded. They trusted Him so they lowered their nets one more time despite having spent the entire night fishing and catching nothing. They abandoned their fear of failing again and chose to trust instead.

How amazing it is when we might contemplate the reality that we are needed; we have something to give that no one else can give, which is ourselves. Despite our misconceptions, doubts, and disbeliefs, we are part of central casting in the realm of life. Each of us has been given a role we never imagined nor could we foresee. The various stages of life have elements of both tragedy and comedy. We have the task and the responsibility to donate whatever we have and whoever we are to someone, anyone who might benefit from our kindness. No matter how weak and wounded we think ourselves to be, God can do wonders with those who choose to be instruments of love. Herein we find the faith to believe and the trust to be vulnerable.

An elderly rabbi once asked his students how they could tell when night had ended and the day had begun.

"Could it be when you see an animal in the distance and can tell whether it is a sheep or a dog?"

"No," answered the rabbi.

"Could it be when you look at a tree in the distance and can tell whether it is a fig tree or a peach tree?"

"No," again the rabbi answered.

"Well, then, when is it?" the students demanded.

"It is when you look on the face of any woman or man and see that she or he is your sister or brother. Because if you cannot do this, then no matter what time it is, it is still night!"

How have we lived in darkness? Blinded by our prejudices and fears, have we failed to see what stands before us, the image of someone with whom we have distanced ourselves? The distance of seeing clearly can be compromised by our own narrow views and opinions. The limited vision of sight and understanding will bring darkness and blindness to our minds as well as our eyes.

There are none so blind that refuse to see. Some may have indeed preferred the darkness more than the light. It's safe there, no doubt, but nothing will ever grow there, except maybe mushrooms.

History is filled with those who did little or nothing to address or confront the injustices and oppression of others. Many felt and believed that the suffering of others was not their concern or their business, yet we know that history has proven otherwise.

"When the Nazis came for the communists,

I remained silent; I was not a communist.

When they locked up the social democrats,

I remained silent; I was not a social democrat.

When they came for the trade unionists,

I did not speak out; I was not a trade unionist.

When they came for the Jews,

I remained silent; I wasn't a Jew.

When they came for me, there was no one left to speak out."

— Martin Niemöller, a Protestant Minister in Germany.

We may do well to examine our own responses to the injustices and suffering of others. What have we said and done to raise our voices and address the issues about the plight of others? Pretending it's not our problem is only one way of stating we don't want to get involved. But as Edmund Burke has written so well, "The only thing necessary for the triumph of evil is that good men do nothing."

Yes, the fear of becoming involved inhibits and stifles our efforts to do good, which is necessary and essential for the survival of humanity in general. We cannot resign ourselves to the false notion we have nothing to offer, nothing to give, and cannot make a difference.

Chapter Seventeen

The Power to Make a Difference

One of my favorite stories I have told and retold throughout my life is the story of an old man walking a Florida beach after a storm. Tossed upon the seashore were various species of marine life, and shells, countless numbers of shells. As the man ambled along the shoreline, he saw in the distance a young boy repeatedly bending down, picking up something, and then tossing it into the ocean. As he came closer, the man noticed the boy was throwing starfish back into the sea. Indeed there were so many littering the beach that it appeared his task was hopeless. The old man watched the boy for several minutes. Finally, he spoke up and asked, "Young man, what are you doing?" Without even bothering to look at the man, the boy said, "Sir, I'm trying to save these starfish!" The man continued to observe the boy's relentless efforts. Finally he asked again, "Boy, what difference can you make? There's only one of you and hundreds of starfish." The boy stopped, looked at the man, and holding a starfish in his hands, he cast it into the ocean and as he did so he said, "It'll make a difference to that one!"

There are times when we look at the enormity of a problem or a challenge and we become paralyzed into inactivity. Somehow we cannot conceive of making a difference on any level. So instead, we do nothing, or very little at all. The premium that is often placed on the quantity of those who will benefit from one's charity is a serious deterrent for some in doing even the smallest acts of goodness. Unless the numbers are impressive, most will not waste their time or efforts, as they see it, to do something substantial for others. Too much of an emphasis has been unfairly placed on "how many" rather than the "who" and the "what." Those we help and what we do have far more significance than the numbers affected.

Of course, the result of helping many is admirable but not all of us have that large an audience nor that enormous potential. We do what we can do because we can; we do for others what we can because ultimately we choose to do so. Sounds simple, eh? It is until we realize there are fears that disconnect us from this reality. To venture out of our comfort zones into the land of risk and possible harm is no small mission for us to pursue.

There is an Indonesian story about a holy man walking along a road when a beggar comes up to him and asks, "Alms for the poor? Alms for the poor?" The holy man turns to the beggar, opens his satchel, and says, "Help yourself, my good man." The beggar looks into the sack and spies a gorgeous jewel, a huge stone, obviously of great value. The beggar instantly knows such a stone will make him enormously wealthy and fixed for life. He grabs the jewel and quickly leaves. Three days later he finds the holy man and says to him, "Excuse me, sir, I would like to return this jewel, as precious as it is, and ask you for something far more precious." The holy man asked, "What is that?" To which the beggar responded, "That which enabled you to give it to me."

How many of us would elect to return this precious jewel for something far more valuable? Do we even accept the fact that the ability to be so generous is indeed more priceless than any amount of material wealth? This is exactly where the crux of our self-fulfillment rests. Here is where we determine the priority of living and giving for ourselves only, or living and giving for the sake of others. There can be no avoidance of this path for our lives, either we do or we don't.

Each of us has the free will and intellect to make decisions that influence and shape our character and personality. Dedicating our minds to learn more of the hardships and afflictions of others is a first step. The second is even more important: when we resolve within ourselves to do something about the plight others are forced to endure.

President Woodrow Wilson once said, "No one can love his neighbor on an empty stomach."

Likewise, it has also been said by the great Colombian saint, Peter Claver, S.J., "Before we can feed their souls, we must feed their stomachs."

Even earlier in time, Cato the Roman Censor said, "An empty stomach has no ears."

Their point is obvious: we are all created with both a body and a soul. Until we minister to the physical needs of the suffering and the needy we can never help them with their other needs. Isn't this exactly what the greatest spiritual leaders throughout history have done in their lives? Eventually more people will be influenced by our expressions of charity than anything we could ever tell them. Our good works will speak so loudly and clearly, it will not be possible to be misunderstood.

Chapter Eighteen

The Consequences of Our Compassion

Whatever good deeds we perform for the benefit of others truly have many unforeseen consequences. Much like all human activity, one can never predict the ripple effect of both good and evil behavior. When we trust a Higher Power, then we can be certain that our kindness and generosity has no end. We can take assurance that whatever we do for those who are in need will far exceed our expectations. Once again, there is the all-important factor of *trust*. If we permit fear to control us, then there will be little hope or conviction that our compassion and benevolence have any chance of expression or survival.

A water bearer in India had two large clay pots, each of which hung on the end of a pole that he carried across the back of his neck. One of the pots had developed a crack in it and the other pot was undamaged. Thus the latter pot always delivered a full portion of water at the end of the long walk from the stream to the master's house, while the cracked pot delivered only half of its portion.

For years, this went on daily, with the water bearer delivering one and a half pots of water to his master's house. Of course, the unbroken pot was proud of its accomplishments, perfect to the end for which it was made. But the poor cracked pot was ashamed of its imperfection and miserable that it was only able to perform half of what it had been created to do. After some time of what it perceived itself to be a bitter failure, the cracked pot spoke to its bearer one day by the stream: "I am so ashamed of myself and I want to apologize to you." The bearer asked, "Why? What are you ashamed of?"

"I have been able for these past few years to deliver only half of my load because of the crack in my side, which causes the water to leak out all the way back to your master's house. Because of this flaw you have to do all of this work and you do not get full value from your efforts," said the pot. The water bearer felt sorry for the old cracked pot and in compassion he said, "As we return to the master's house I want you to notice the beautiful flowers along the path." Indeed as they went up the hill, the cracked pot noticed the sun warming the beautiful flowers on the side of the path. But at the end of the path, the pot felt sad because once again, half of its load was missing and so it once again apologized to its bearer for its failure.

The bearer said to the pot, "Did you notice that there were flowers on only one side of the path but not on the other side? That's because I have always known about your flaw and I sought to use it for good. I planted flower seeds on that side of the path and every day when we walked back from the stream to the master's house, you watered them. For years now, I have been able to pick these flowers to decorate my master's table. Without you being just the way you are, he would never have had this beauty to grace his house.

Few of us could ever conceive of such magnificent consequences for one's act of rescue and subsequent healing. The irony of life seems to be this: the more we seek to understand its mysteries, the more it astounds us, the mysteries we continuously uncover. As Graham Greene said so eloquently, "I would never believe in a God I could understand."

To be content with unanswered questions, with mysteries that abound and surround us, to acknowledge our powerlessness and our ever present fears, is to begin to see *love* as the only way in which to find peace and fulfillment in life. Choosing to be tied to unanswered questions, allowing ourselves to be controlled by our fears, and never risking the opportunity to be vulnerable are recipes for an unhappy and miserable life.

We have the power to choose, to decide whether we want to live or to begin to die. Our choice of a slow death, succumbing to the fears we enable within us, most certainly will imperil our future, our health, and wellbeing.

We cannot avoid such tragic results when we consent to the power of the fears that strive to control us. To love is to let go of one's fears.

As the great Jesuit theologian, Pierre Telhard de Chardin, once said: "Someday, after mastering the winds, the waves, the tides, and gravity, we shall harness for God the energies of love, and then for the second time in the history of the world, man will discover fire."

Chapter Nineteen

Our Priorities Help Define Us

Each of us is wounded; let's accept that as fact. We will never move beyond our self-loathing and self-pity until we recognize and accept this reality. Yet our wounds can be a tremendous source of understanding, sympathy, and compassion, more importantly, *love*. When we no longer view our wounds as obstacles or sources of embarrassment, then we can welcome them into our personality as indispensable gifts. We are not destined to be in this world without the purpose and promise of leaving behind a legacy that can transform the life of even one person. We each have a purpose. No matter how seemingly small or insignificant, we have the potential and capacity to assist another to discover their true selves and their unrecognized talents.

The following words from a fourteen-year-old girl might be too idealistic and naïve in the opinion of some but I encourage you to read them and reflect on them: "Everyone has inside himself a piece of good news. The good news is that you really don't know how great you can be, how much you can love, what you can accomplish, and what your potential is. How can you top good news like that?"

Some adults might consider such thoughts as too optimistic but when you learn the author of those words, you might well be surprised. Her name was Anne Frank. Millions upon millions of people have read her diary narrating her experiences as she and her family hid from the Nazis. Her story survived and has become a testimony to the human spirit. Anne's diary will continue to be read as long as human beings struggle to survive in a world tarnished by despair, corrupted by madness, and degenerated by savagery.

Yes, there is within all of us potential that remains to be discovered, developed, and realized. Until we ignite the fire of self-discovery, we shall remain in the darkness of who we are and what we can do. Life is a series of trials, filled with success and error. The experience of both helps determine our unique talents, abilities, and passions. Every day we have the opportunity to sift through the endless possibilities of our potential, probing them, wearing them, and trying them on as one would a new pair of shoes... How do they fit? How do they look? How do they feel?

There is an old German city called Weinsberg. The city rests on a high hill overlooking a valley below. Atop the hill enclosing the city is an ancient fortress. The people who live in Weinsberg speak of a fascinating legend about their city. During the fifteenth century, a time of chivalry and honor, an enemy encircled the city and sealed off escape. The leader of the enemy force sent word to those in the fortress that all the women and the children would be spared and find freedom. The women would be permitted to take with them their most valuable possessions if they could carry it upon their backs. This was the type of chivalrous conduct and word of honor that was both given and known for this time in history. You can well imagine the shock and consternation when the enemies and their leader watched the women exit the fortress, each carrying her husband on her back.

What is it we most treasure in life? Is it someone we love? Is it our rank, position, or status? Maybe it is our health or our personal achievements. Whatever it is we value the most, we carry it through life, the burden can be light or it can be heavy.

The weight may well depend on whether the value of what we hold nearest and dearest truly contributes to our wellbeing or not. The more fulfilling and noble the treasure, then the lighter the weight of its bearing. Whatever we carry in our hearts or bear upon our backs is much lighter when it is accepted and embraced as a gift or a life lesson rather than a burden or source of suffering.

Chapter Twenty

Controlling Our Concept of God

This chapter can be the most frightening. Why? Because it challenges us to abandon our desire to control what we have been told we could control from our earliest years of religious instruction. In effect, it's very much like being told, "There is no Santa Claus!"

Throughout history, humans have sought to understand, to know, and to appease the forces beyond them. The search for the Divine is but one of these. Civilizations have come and gone which have endeavored to express their worship of an All-Powerful and All-Knowing One. Whether from a polytheistic approach or a monotheistic one, humanity has an innate need to find its Origin. It can be said that to think and speak theologically, is to speak and think what is fundamentally human. Many have sought to write about God, speak about Him, preach and teach about Him, but the ability to fix or to control God is fruitless. These attempts, as Abraham Heschel has put it, are as successful as trying to fly an airplane made of stone.

The renowned Russian writer Leo Tolstoy once wrote: "If the thought comes to you that everything that you have thought about God is mistaken and that there is no God, do not be dismayed. It happens to many people. But do not think that the source of your unbelief is that there is no God. If you no longer believe in the God in whom you believed before, this comes from the fact that there is something wrong with your belief, and you must strive to grasp better that which you call God. When a savage ceases to believe in his wooden God, this does not mean that there is no God, but that the true God is not of wood."

This very insightful and wise statement from Tolstoy may seem to most of us to have no personal application to our lives because we have never believed in gods made of wood or any other such primitive idols, but then we would miss the point entirely. We may not believe in a god of wood but we do believe in one of our own making and imaging, one we think will grant us what we want and answer all our prayers. When this concept of the god we have fashioned does not prove to be real and does not hear our prayers, then we begin to lose faith in God altogether. Most definitely, it is easy to lose faith in a god who allows us to suffer great pain and torment. Remember the words of St. Paul in regards to our understanding of faith in God: "When I was a child, I used to speak like a child, think like a child, reason like a child, when I became a man, I did away with childish things." 1Corinthians 13:11-12.

Unfortunately, there are many of us whose image and understanding of God is still as wooden and as primitive as ever. It hasn't changed since our childhood. No wonder many so-called "religious" people still view God in such a childlike fashion. How many still conceive of the Divine as some sort of Santa Claus, or the Wizard of Oz? Some believe in a god who grants requests when called upon to do so, dispensing favorable responses based on one's sincerity and righteous efforts. These people have kept their vision of god fixed in a form and understanding which no longer conforms to their own maturation in life. They may have matured in some areas of their life but their spiritual life was not one of them.

In some cultures and religions, the portrait or image of someone, especially the Divine, is strictly forbidden. Photographing or depicting the picture or appearance of an individual for some persons is absolutely prohibited. Some maintain that capturing such a pictorial manifestation steals one's "spirit." In some religions, like Islam, Eastern Orthodox Christianity, and others, certain likenesses of the Divine are strictly banned. Even in Judaism the regulations for written expressions of G-d are clearly made evident.

How many religious denominations practice the use of objects or rituals to influence God? How many so-called "faith-filled" people wear medals, scapulars, carry rosaries and other religious items as amulets to protect themselves from accident, injury, or danger? Those who do so employ a usage of religious emblems and practices which quite frankly manifest more of a belief in magic than trust. Isn't this what magic essentially means? The controlling of nature or spirits. When people are fearful they will no doubt succumb to any methods to control the threats to their safety or influence the outcomes they desire. No matter how many St. Christopher medals you have in your automobile, they will not prevent you from an accident. Denis Diderot wrote in 1746: "Superstition is more injurious to God than atheism."

The concept of controlling God is regarded as anathema in both Judaism and Islam, for some Christians however, it is not so disallowed.

Consider the doctrine of impassibility. This teaching suggests that God is totally incapable of any emotion, He is incapable of suffering, joy, pain, disappointment, pleasure, happiness, etc. Essentially, the doctrine states that since God is omnipotent, omniscient, all-powerful, and immutable, therefore, He cannot be subject to the same emotions that human beings experience. Since emotions are so fickle and so irregular, the nature of God could not be such, because then He would be subject to change, and He would not be God.

Your first response may be to recall the countless instances in both the Old and New Testaments when the biblical writers employed anthropomorphic descriptions of the Divine reactions and responses. We read about an "angry, vengeful, and even violent God." We read throughout Scripture the attempts by many authors to make God "more human." All that we truly know of God is derived from our imagination. For if we truly knew God as He is, then we would be His equal. Essentially, to know God completely is impossible, or He would not be God.

The belief that we have the ability to please or disappoint God has been a consistent error for some in their religious understanding of the Divine for centuries. God's emotions are nonexistent because God is immutable. He cannot change from happiness to sadness or vice versa. Furthermore, if we had the power to influence or affect the Divine so easily because of our behavior or the lack thereof, He would not be God.

This is a very difficult reality for many who call themselves religious to embrace and accept. Why? Because many are still in the stage of a moral conviction that their good behavior deserves reward and their immoral behavior will be a cause for punishment. Thus we would have the capacity to influence God's favor or not. The concept of a God who rewards and punishes is very primitive and juvenile. Closely allied with this erroneous impression is the belief that we can influence or control God's intervention in human existence.

In the history of human interaction with one or more "Higher Powers" we have found cultures that used their own "religious" practices, words, and rituals for a variety of reasons. Some sought to placate the "volcano god" with the sacrifice of a virgin. Still others sought to appease the gods of agriculture, weather, and war by the human sacrifice of their own tribal members or the lives of their captured enemies. If the sacrifices were not human, then they may have been the offerings of some valuable possession of the petitioner or tribe. Recall the offerings of Cain and Abel: one was the sacrifice of an animal, the other the harvest of one's crops.

Each of these ritualistic observances and practices were attempts to seek favor for the petitioners. Whatever may have been an impending natural disaster or need, or something as simple as a successful hunt are clear signs of the conviction that people thought their "prayers and acts of petition" could influence or change the mind and activity of their god or gods. Greek mythology is rife with such examples. If we could so easily affect God by such rituals and words, then He would not be God.

Imagine if you will, and that is what we always do in regards to the Divine, that two different or opposing groups are praying to the same God for victory, profit, or gain. To whom does God grant His favor?

I realize some of you may recite the words of Jesus in the Gospels of Matthew 7:7 and Luke 11:9: "Ask and it will be given you, seek and you will find, knock and the door will be opened to you. For everyone who asks receives; he who seeks finds; and to him who knocks, the door will be opened."

There isn't any one of us who hasn't wanted God to do something, whether it be to help us, others, or to prevent some possible disaster or crisis. We pray for protection, we pray for good weather, we pray for the health of others. In fact, there isn't much we don't pray that God will influence and intercede for us with His all-powerful presence. Thus, when we read that "if we ask, we shall receive," if "we seek, we shall find," and if "we knock, the door will be opened," this does not mean we'll get the answer we want, nor will we find what we seek nor that door that opens is the one we desired. The only promise we are given is that when we do ask, seek, and knock, we will *always* get a response, just not necessarily the one we wanted. If we *always* received the response we wanted, not only would it be impossible, He would not be God.

Now we return to the beginning of our journey. We must, sooner or later in our lives, accept that there will *always* be questions: Why did this happen? Why didn't God hear my prayer? What did I do wrong? Once again, we return to the suggestion, "everything happens for a reason." This is where we discover either we trust God or we don't.

Matthew 6:25: "...I tell you, do not worry about your life, what you will eat or drink; or about your body, what you will wear, is not life more than food, and the body more than clothes? Look at the birds of the air, they do not sow or reap, or gather into barns, and yet your heavenly Father feeds them. Are you not much more valuable than they?"

The question we cannot avoid now confronts us: Do you trust God to give you what you truly need or don't you? Notice I did not write, what you want. Psalm 22 or 23, depending on your Bible states: "The Lord is my shepherd, there is nothing I shall want."

Really? If this is true, if this is something you recite, believe, and trust, then why, oh why, do you ask God for anything? Do you trust God *always* to give you what you need? It's a yes or no question.

We come to the critical question, the one posed by the high wire artist to the so-called faith-filled spectator: "Are we willing to get into the wheelbarrow?" Hey, it's quite easy to believe in a body of religious doctrines, on the other hand, trusting in someone, anyone, especially God, requires a personal risk that makes us vulnerable. It is a surrender of our control. We abandon the notion that anything we do, any act of piety or devotion is incapable of pleasing God. Eventually, we accept the fact that there is *nothing, absolutely nothing we can do to please God; if we could, He would not be God.* Whatever words or prayers of petition we utter will likewise be for naught. Thus, we can remove the bumper sticker stating that God is our copilot and then we can assume that role.

Prayer is not intended to change the world; it is intended to change us. Then we change the world by the manner in which we look at it. We change our attitudes through prayer and reflection. Then and only then do we change our mindset, or actions and reactions to life in general. Our concept of the world changes before our eyes. What we once perceived in a cynical, sarcastic, and evil manner is changed. Our change of attitude does in reality change the world as we see it. The world remains as it always was and always will be, yet now our perception is transformed.

I maintain the *only* prayers of any merit and worth are prayers we offer to God in thanksgiving, contrition, and adoration. We need to express our gratitude to the Divine, as well as our contrition for our weaknesses and sinfulness. Our manifestations of worship are truly necessary and beneficial, not to God but for the benefit of our own wellbeing, spiritual and otherwise.

Reluctantly, we come to the realization that God does *not* need our prayers. However, He beckons us to be ourselves; He calls us to reflect "the image and likeness in which we were created." God challenges us to reflect His divinity within us.

This is not so much a need of God's but a "calling." A calling to be our real selves, an invitation to become what we are destined to be: One with Him. This is our true vocation in life, to reflect the "image and likeness" of our Creator. We must in the words of Shakespeare, "to our own selves be true." We cannot escape the summons to be co-creators in this world, whatever we do to restore justice, to demonstrate love and forgiveness, is indeed the work of God. We have the shared Divine capacity to heal, restore, and to redeem.

Finally, there can be no true peace and happiness for any of us who seek to control others, events, and God. We will most assuredly fail on all counts. Until we surrender the desire for control, we will meet with disaster and disappointment on a frequent basis. When the day finally dawns upon us that we can only control our actions and responses, then we will have made the transition from fear to trust. We will allow God to be in control; we will trust that He will *always* have our best interest and welfare at heart. Why? We will know Him to be a God who is *love*.

A *love* that is not simply an emotion, but rather one that is a decision, an act of the will, one that is unconditional and eternal. This is not just faith; it is much more, it is *trust*. For *fear* and *love* can never coexist in any relationship.

Chapter Twenty-One

When Religion Seeks to Control

If you think the previous chapter was unsettling, this one will cause even more consternation... Why? Simply because one of the most important roles that religion plays in our society is to offer formation, purpose, healing, and comfort, as well as a moral compass. Yet, as we have become more educated, we have grown to question some of the long-held beliefs we learned early in life. We have witnessed religious hypocrisy on a much wider scale. We have seen betrayal by religious leaders who were all too weak to admit their own failures. We came to see, "the emperor had no clothes."

The renowned Jewish philosopher, Abraham Heschel, in his book, *God in Search of Man,* wrote: "It is customary to blame secular science and anti-religious philosophy for the eclipse of religion in modern society. It would be more honest to blame religion for its own defeats. Religion declined not because it was refuted, but because it became irrelevant, dull, oppressive, insipid. When faith is completely replaced by creed, worship by discipline, love by habit; when the crisis of today is ignored because of the splendor of the past; when faith becomes an heirloom rather than a living fountain; when religion speaks only in the name of authority rather than with the voice of compassion — its message becomes meaningless."

What profound insights these are by such a deeply spiritual man. Remi De Roo, the former Catholic bishop of Victoria makes similar comments. When there were those who commented to him regarding their concerns about the future of the Church, De Roo responded: "The worst is yet to come." He advised his listeners, "Don't get lost in intellectual battles... if you think carefully of what Vatican II said, it reminds us very clearly that our baptismal vocation is primarily oriented to society, not to the Church. The Church is not an end in itself. The Church is only an instrument for the promotion of the reign of God... The fundamental mission of Jesus was not to build a Church (but)... to proclaim the reign of God. The primary mission of the baptized was not ministry in the Church... It is the proclaiming of the reign of God throughout the whole cosmos in whatever sphere that happens to be, whether it is astronomy, literature, politics, music, dancing."

We can never forget, the Church exists not as a society of the righteous and the worthy but rather in the words of Charles Clayton Morrison: "The Christian Church is a society of sinners. It is the only society in the world in which membership is based on the single qualification that the candidate be unworthy of membership."

Elton Trueblood, the Quaker scholar wrote this: "True religion is not man's search for the good life, important as that may be. Neither is it our effort to find God, inevitable as that may be. True religion is our response to Him who seeks us. It is not an argument for God, but a response to God's love."

More recently, Pope Francis has called the Church "...a field hospital after battle. It is useless to ask a seriously injured person if he has high cholesterol and about the level of his blood sugars. You have to heal his wounds. Then we can talk about everything else."

Sometimes organized religion has sought to control how people think, and we know all too well it also seeks to control how its members act.

It was Bertrand Russell who said, "Religion is based, I think, primarily and mainly upon fear."

Organized religions have sought to portray themselves as sole proprietors of *truth*, as means to further control and exercise their influence. Such a claim to the provenance of *truth* was addressed by John L. Allen, Jr. in "Faith, Hope and Heroes," National Catholic Reporter, February 23, 2001: "It is my conviction that humanity can only exist in the plural. As soon as we claim to possess the truth or speak in the name of humanity we fall into totalitarianism and exclusion. No one possesses the truth; everyone seeks it."

The word "religion" comes from the Latin word "religare" that means "to bind." There are many times when religion endeavors to bind, control, and manipulate, often under the pretext that it is in the interest of "saving" the individual. Unlike Michelangelo, it does not always see the capacity for potential and the inherent beauty within its subjects. Sometimes institutional religious bodies employ *fear* as a means to command its flock to comply with their rules, regulations, and laws, rather than the higher motive of *love*. According to some, failing to adhere to these religiously established norms, puts one's afterlife at risk. Using *fear* as a means to control seems far more effective than *love*. The fears of going to hell, eternal damnation, or separation from the Divine have been traditionally used as such threats. Taught by some religions for centuries as a means to regulate the actions and beliefs of their adherents.

No one can deny the need for order through discipline and rules in both religious and civil societies. No one can deny the necessity of law, but the primacy of love supersedes it. However, there have been countless scenes in the history of religions that the *means* has become more important than the *end*. Wherein the *law* has been elevated to a status that becomes idolized, when the "Letter of the Law" is more important than the "Spirit of the Law."

The Scottish theologian, William Barclay, tells the story of an imprisoned rabbi in the city of Rome. He was given minimal rations of food and water. Time would pass and the rabbi grew weaker and weaker. Eventually, a doctor was called and the rabbi was diagnosed as being severely dehydrated. The jailers could not understand why their prisoner had become so dehydrated. Even though he was given the minimum of water, he still had no reason to be so weak. After the doctor's visit, the guards were instructed to observe their prisoner closely, which they did. They then discovered why the rabbi was so dehydrated. He was using all the water given to him to perform his religious ritual washings prior to his prayer and meal, thus he had nothing left to drink.

The rituals that are often performed in organized religion are designed to be a means to an end; they are not ends in themselves. What truly is significant in religious devotion is not what we do, but *why* we do it. Whenever we elevate the rituals to such a status, we give more importance to the actions and not the intentions. Very much like Kohlberg's theory of moral development, one's intentions to obey, to do good, or to follow one's religious convictions are the critical factors in determining moral maturity. H. L. Mencken said it best: "Morality is doing what's right no matter what you are told. Religion is doing what you are told, no matter what is right."

Confusion has long reigned in organized religion when it places far too much emphasis on ritual practices and not on the motive of the worshipper. To help someone purify his or her intentions is the call to act in love, a higher motive and not for a lesser one.

A further example of this unfortunate mistake in religious observance is a quote by the Presbyterian minister Spencer Marsh who once said the following: "A warning notice should be written on the cover of every Bible: 'The intent of this book is always to point to the God who loves you. Do not allow it to become an end in itself. That would be idolatry.'"

How many biblical literalists and fundamentalists would recoil at such an admonition?

Whenever we mistake the "means" for the "end," it is then that we lose sight of the reason for our religious worship. The means becomes our idol, a fault that was most evident in the Pharisees' over-emphasis on the law. How many of us recognize such religious legalism today? Some congregants see themselves as defenders of the faith, militants, if you will, when in actuality they are only asked to be witnesses of it.

Organized religion has been responsible for some heinous and less than credible teachings and actions in history. Consider for a moment these edicts from the Catholic Church.

This statement is from the Papal Bull, "Cantate Domino" by Pope Eugene IV during the Council of Florence in 1438-1445: "It (the Catholic Church) firmly believes, professes, and proclaims that those not living within the Catholic Church, not only pagans, but also Jews and heretics and schismatics cannot become participants in eternal life, but will depart into everlasting fire which was prepared for the devil and his angels [Matt. 25:41], unless before the end of life the same have been added to the flock; and that the unity of the ecclesiastical body is so strong that only to those remaining in it are the sacraments of the Church of benefit for salvation, and do fastings, almsgiving, and other functions of piety and exercises of Christian service produce eternal reward, and that no one, whatever almsgiving he has practiced, even if he has shed blood for the name of Christ, can be saved, unless he has remained in the bosom and unity of the Catholic Church."

Or this one from Pope Boniface, the Papal Bull, "Unam Sanctam" in 1302: "Indeed we declare, say, pronounce, and define that it is altogether necessary to salvation for every human creature to be subject to the Roman Pontiff."

And finally, from Pope Innocent III, during the Fourth Lateran Council, 1215: "One indeed is the universal Church of the faithful, outside which no one at all is saved."

Teachings such as those above, became a subtle means to eliminate those who did not share the faith of the Church. Indirectly, those outside the faith were viewed as undesirables and thus excluded not only from activities and rights in this life but the next as well. One can only imagine the cruelty many endured, all in the name of God.

Thankfully, the Catholic Church modified the belief "extra ecclesiam nulla salus" translated, "there is no salvation outside the Church." During Vatican II, the document, "Lumen Gentium" was issued by Pope Paul VI in 1964 which clearly refutes the previous papal edicts about salvation in chapter 16:

[16] "Finally, those who have not yet received the Gospel are related to the People of God in various ways.

"There is, first, that people to which the covenants and promises were made, and from which Christ was born according to the flesh (cf. Rom. 9:4-5): in view of the divine choice, they are a people most dear for the sake of the fathers, for the gifts of God are without repentance (cf. Rom. 11:29-29). But the plan of salvation also includes those who acknowledge the Creator, in the first place amongst whom are the Moslems: these profess to hold the faith of Abraham, and together with us they adore the one, merciful God, mankind's judge on the last day. Nor is God remote from those who in shadows and images seek the unknown God, since he gives to all men life and breath and all things (cf. Acts 17:25-28), and since the Saviour wills all men to be saved (cf. 1 Tim. 2:4). Those who, through no fault of their own, do not know the Gospel of Christ or his Church, but who nevertheless seek God with a sincere heart, and, moved by grace, try in their actions to do his will as they know it through the dictates of their conscience — those too may achieve eternal salvation.

"Nor shall divine providence deny the assistance necessary for salvation to those who, without any fault of theirs, have not yet arrived at an explicit knowledge of God, and who, not without grace, strive to lead a good life."

So much for the belief that there is no salvation outside the Church!

This change in doctrine came after centuries of theological development, and like all changes, it was slow and tedious, seemingly bordering on theological hubris. To claim that this branch of Christianity was a means not only to control others but likewise it also claimed to control God. Recall the earlier story I cited about those who could not accept an all-merciful and all-loving God, one that could forgive anyone and admit sinners to eternal life. For those law-biding and religiously narrow-minded individuals, it was absolutely inconceivable for God to be so unconditionally loving.

Unfortunately, religion does like to impose conditions, not just for this world but for the next as well. There is, for instance, a history of religious conflict fraught with atrocities and brutality that continue to amaze and bewilder us. Blaise Pascal said: "Men never commit evil so fully and joyfully as when they do it for religious convictions."

When the marriage of religion and nationalism is wrought, it can be a particularly toxic brand of "fanaticism." There are those who are willing to give their lives in service of their country, still more are willing to offer their lives in service to both their religion and their country. Such a marriage produces some of the worst evil perpetrated on humanity.

In the Old Testament, the concept of "herem" is such an example of the worst forms of human immorality. According to Deuteronomy 7:1-2; Deuteronomy 20:16-18; 1 Samuel 15:1-3, every enemy of the Israelites, man, woman, and child, was to be killed and shown no mercy. Even the crops and cattle were destroyed and no spoils of victory were permitted for the conquerors. More so, the victorious Israelites were instructed to salt the land of their enemies so that nothing would ever grow there for years.

This appears like genocide, doesn't it? Such destruction and annihilation of a people does not seem like a genuine reflection of G-d, does it? More than anything, it appears to be a human mandate for the Israelite warfare and subjugation of its enemies.

The Armenian Genocide by the Ottoman Turks from 1915 to the early 1920s is yet another example of one religious group inflicting the near systematic massacre of another people because of their ethnicity and religious persuasion. The Caucasus region had been inhabited for over 3,000 years and it is believed by some that Armenia was the first nation in history to proclaim

Christianity as its national religion. The Turks killed an estimated 1.5 million Armenians because they sought to have only one nationality and one religion in the empire.

We could easily recount the horrors inflicted by the Crusaders on the so-called infidels and vice versa. Such brutality was easily dismissed for its "religious" purposes.

One particularly gruesome scene that was recorded in Catholic Church history happened at the siege of Malta by the Turks in 1565. The threat of the Turks to Europe was real; the entire Mediterranean Sea was becoming a Turkish lake. The Turkish fleet numbered 200 vessels. The fortress at Malta was being defended by several hundred of the Knights of St. John under the command of Jean Parisot de La Valette, their Grand Master. Valette was once offered the position of cardinal, Prince of the Church, but declined the position.

The leader of the Turkish fleet was Mustapha Pasha. His contempt for the Christian faith was so deep that he had the heads of four knights who had been captured, decapitated and their bodies nailed to crosses in mockery of the crucifixion. When the currents of the Mediterranean waters surrounding Malta brought the bodies of the knights to the foot of the great fortress, Valette saw clearly the meaning of this act. This was a "guerre a la outrance": a "war with no quarter."

In response to Pasha's brutality, Valette sent a message of his own. He directed all the Turkish prisoners be brought to the ramparts and there they would be beheaded. He then ordered the severed heads be placed into the fort's cannons and fired into the Turkish positions. We shake our heads in utter disbelief at the atrocities and horrific acts that are still part of our modern world. History clearly shows that nothing is new under the sun; it demonstrates we have not tempered our zeal to dehumanize our enemy, even under the most "religious" banner and battle-inspiring slogans of misdirected faith.

This loss of credibility and respect have been a slow erosive dynamic that has undermined the foundation of what we had long invested our deepest trust and convictions. Nowadays, people seem to prefer to identify themselves as "spiritual" rather than "religious." It has been said, some people are religious because of their fear of hell, others are spiritual because they have already been through hell.

All too many have accepted the fact that one "body of religion" does not have all the answers, some of whose answers appear ridiculous and impossible. Instead of helping humanity, quite often religion has been a major source of its pain and suffering.

One of the most egregious periods of Catholic history has been the sexual abuse crisis of the last half-century around the world. While this type of abuse has been part of the Church's history for centuries, it did not become fully apparent until the secular media committed itself to uncovering the pervasive extent of these horrible crimes, the lies and concealment regarding them. The ecclesiastical leaders unfortunately obscured the real facts. In doing so, they also compromised the highest value: truth. Their priorities were skewed. Fear will do that.

Equally astounding is this fact: it was not until 1965 that the Catholic Church officially and universally condemned any and all forms of slavery in "Gaudium et Spes," chapter 29. What did Abraham Lincoln know in 1863 that the Church didn't?

In 1992, Pope John Paul II apologized for the Catholic Church's treatment of Galileo Galilei. In so doing, the pope set a precedent that many popes had the opportunity to perform but failed to do so. Galileo dared to teach that the universe was heliocentric and not geocentric, a theory previously proposed by Copernicus. The Church refused to accept such a position. According to the Catholic Church, the earth was the center of the universe and not the sun. Galileo was sentenced to house arrest and charged with heresy for his refusal to change his scientific beliefs. He eventually died at age seventy-seven, nine years after his "informal imprisonment" began.

This same pope also begged forgiveness from Muslims, Jews, and those who perished during the Crusades and later the Inquisition. Much to his credit, this pope was willing to own and embrace the Church's sins and seek forgiveness. What has most polarized those who belong to some congregations against their institutional church is the failure or reluctance of today's "religious" leaders to do the same.

We have become aware of various television evangelists whose secretive lifestyle has been anything but exemplary or honest. We know there are those who "often protest too much." In time, their wounds and the weaknesses become all too obvious.

When fear dominates the thinking and management of any organization, then the tactics from such direction will reduce the integrity and character of that same body. As Lucretius said, "Fear is the mother of all gods." In the final analysis, we realize those "gods" are false. We have been worshipping at the wrong altar.

This brings me to a final point. As I mentioned, humans have struggled throughout history to find the Divine. They have sought to control God, possess God, and use God. The Ark of the Covenant is but one example. Look at the purpose of the Crusades: to recover the Holy Land from the "infidels." To this day, one of the most sacred sites for the three major religions,

Judaism, Christianity, and Islam is the Dome of the Rock in Jerusalem. Here each of the three major religions believe a sacred event occurred. For the Jews and for Christians it is believed to be the location of Abraham's aborted attempt to sacrifice his son Isaac. For Muslims, it is believed to be the place where Muhammad ascended into heaven accompanied by the angel Gabriel.

Localizing God is once again further evidence of our futile attempts to control the Divine. God is everywhere, or He would not be God.

When Jesus Christ declared, "Wherever two or more are gathered in my name, I am in their midst" (Matthew 18:19), Jesus essentially removed the possibility of the Divine being confined and localized.

Today, however, there are many places that are believed to hold a sacred Presence: the Wailing Wall, church buildings, temples and mosques of all denominations, Mecca, the Vatican, Varanasi/Kashi, Bodhgaya, etc. While these holy sites have a religious significance, they can never replace the value of a human life. They are merely a means to an end, not the end in itself. These are signposts: they can for some pilgrims, point the way, but they can never be misconstrued as *the* way. The way or path is revealed in the witness of those who live and act in the Spirit of Love.

Every other path will ultimately lead to ruin.

Regrettably, the misguided attempts to protect the safety of churches, houses, shrines, and places of worship have come at the cost of many human lives. We have misplaced our priorities, in protecting buildings, structures, and places we have allowed others to perish in the name of protecting religion. That is indeed sad, because instead of being the path for others to follow, the path itself has been lost or compromised. In the abandonment of trust, fear has ruled the minds and hearts of those who were leaders in faith. In seeking to protect the body of faith, they sacrificed its heart and soul.

Chapter Twenty-Two

What All Religions Can Teach Us

I would like to bring this part of our journey to a conclusion. Throughout human history and its various religious denominations, many have sought to capture the essential truths of human interaction with each other and with a Divine Being. Each has expressed the Golden Rule in one manner or another, always placing the emphasis on what is right, what is just, and what is most loving. Any other rules, mandates, dictums, and teachings pale in comparison. There is no greater act than to treat another as you wish to be treated.

Until the religions of the world focus on the core of their message, they will flounder in their work. Unless religions are willing to build bridges, walls will separate and divide them, one from the other. As long as some religions preach salvation as a gift restricted only to their membership, then there will acrimony, suspicion, and distrust, one for the other. Eventually, in cooperation with the Divine, humanity will either learn to respect each other's beliefs and differences, or they will perish. In time, hopefully all those who call themselves religious will recognize that only *love* can be both their message and their method.

It is no accident that the so-called Golden Rule exists in some form in all the major religions of the world.

Christianity: "In everything, therefore, treat people the same way you want them to treat you, for this is the Law and the Prophets." Matthew 7:12

Judaism: "What is hateful to you, do not to your fellowmen. That is the entire Torah; all the rest is commentary." Talmud, Shabbat, 31a

Islam: "No one of you is a believer until he desires for his brother that which he desires for himself." Sunnah

Brahmanism/Hinduism: "This is the sum of duty: Do naught unto others which would cause you pain if done to you." Mahabharata, 5, 1517

Confucianism: "Surely it is the maxim of loving kindness: Do not unto others that you should not have them do unto you." Analect 15, 23

Buddhism: "Hurt not others in ways that you yourself would find hurtful." Udana-Varga, 5, 18

Taoism: "Regard your neighbor's gain as your gain, and your neighbor's loss as your loss." T'ai Shang Kan Yink P'ien

Zoroastrianism: "That nature alone is good which refrains from doing unto another whatsoever is not good for itself." Dadistan-i-dinik, 94, 5

How curious it is, the simple logic of such teachings are accepted, taught, and believed by all these religions. But the significance does not consist in what is taught or believed. The real significance exists when believers becomes doers, when belief becomes a lifestyle. Therein lies a world of difference. We would never be able to do such great things in our lives unless God loved us so much. For this source of *love* assures us that despite our human foibles and sinfulness, nothing can separate us from Him, a life-changing discovery that begs to be shared with others.

True and honest self-acceptance, the admission and ownership of one's faults and sins, is a humbling act; one that also permits us to see others who have the same issues with a more compassionate attitude. We change what we can control, namely the attitudes we possess that have caused so much hurtful judgment and division on our behalf.

When those who accept, embrace, and own their fears and weaknesses for the sake of saving others, then this much is certain, those doing the saving of the needy, in the process save themselves as well. This is primarily the message and mission of religion itself, or else it would not be from God.

Rejoice in your wounds and afflictions; otherwise, you could not do what you could for those in need, not even the angels could do what you could do. Eventually, we come to understand and accept in life, that only the wounded can be of authentic service to God and others.

Epilogue

A good friend of mine, who previewed the manuscript for this book, encouraged me to include a personal testimony. As I mentioned before, becoming more transparent and vulnerable is a lifelong endeavor. Just when one thinks that he or she has exposed their deepest and darkest secrets, there appears more to be revealed.

My own personal experiences have helped me formulate some of the questions, ideas, and insights that have been presented in this text. I never could have discussed these topics without the essential element of personal involvement. Like you, I am all too familiar with those who talk a good talk but have little contact with the subject matter. For that reason, and others as well, I have chosen to pose some practical questions and examples that open us to greater understanding of the mystery of being human.

Having been ordained a Catholic priest thirty-nine years ago, after spending twelve years in seminary formation and education, I was assigned to a parish for the first two years of my ministry. In the following years I would teach, preach, and serve the People of God in various capacities. During those years I encountered both the worst and the best of humanity, the saddest and the happiest, the most compassionate and the cruelest, the most honest and the most hypocritical. Any and all of these could easily ensure that one might become a cynic. To face the reality that exposes dreams and ideals as being false and filled with pretense is the foundational earthquake of one's life, true game changers. Just as one discovers that his or her relationship is unreal, imagined, or dishonest, so too did I discover that my priestly vocation and the virtues and values on which it was founded were too idealistic and too unauthentic.

The decision to retire from active ministry brought numerous reactions and responses from others to my change of life. Telephone calls, correspondence, and other forms of communication that once received an immediate or timely response went without reply or explanation. Invitations to events, both personal and professional, were no longer extended. Essentially, the step from the pedestal to the ground floor was far greater than I had anticipated.

Few positions in life assure one, as they once did, of immediate respect when one is a priest. To most, he is admired and esteemed for various reasons. Unfortunately, as recent history has clearly exposed, priesthood is no longer deserving of the unquestioned regard and deference it once held. It was during this time of newsworthy exposés that the general public became aware of the ugliness of what occurred behind the rectory and chancery doors. Furthermore, the subsequent denials, obfuscation, and outright lies led even the most ardent Catholic to be scandalized and questioning of his or her faith.

In this time of deep examination and personal reflection, I began my slow transition from being in service to the institution to being in service to my conscience. The trip was neither simple nor short. Inside, I was keenly aware I may not need to live with others but I had to live with myself, and until I did so, I would never be at peace, nor would I ever be happy.

Confronting my family and loved ones with my determined spirit to free myself was the most challenging of all. Vicariously, my parents had lived their lives through me; to some lesser degree, so did my siblings. When I was asked why I was making such a move, it was my own happiness that was paramount. One member of my family suggested that my leaving would make them unhappy. My reply was direct: I was not in charge of their happiness.

All too often we allow ourselves to be held captive by another's happiness or peace of mind. In short, we permit others to control our lives because we do not want to disappoint them or make them unhappy. For too long there had been a simmering anger and intense dislike toward those I felt imprisoning me. Once I came to the realization that I was giving them permission to do so, I knew I had to take back my own life. I had to confront those to whom I had surrendered my free will and self-determination. I had to look my fear right in the face.

The pain and disappointment that family and friends felt over my initial decision linger to this day. I cannot be responsible or in charge of their feelings nor can I assuage them. In my departure from priestly ministry I did make a wonderful discovery: I found my truest and dearest friends. Their relationship with me was not based on what I was, or what I could do for them, rather it was built on who I was to them. Such a profound and eye-opening revelation only further convinced me that I had chosen the path to better understanding and peace.

Through these past sixty-five years of my life, I have been both blessed and challenged. Living a full life does demand the acceptance of both the joy and pain, the good and the bad, successes and losses, the accomplishments and the embarrassments. Suffice it to say, like you, I have had my share of both sides of living.

I can attest to this insight that has slowly, ever more clearly shown itself to be true and valuable to me, that is, the quality of one's friendships are without a price. My own experience with the friendships that have not stood the test of time, or those that have ended in misunderstanding or worse, betrayal, have become all too enlightening. Having been the subject of front-page stories, editorials, false allegations, accusations, and litigation, I continue to struggle with forgiveness.

Thus, when I have written of the necessity of such an act, I do not do so from a purely pedagogical perspective, I do so from one who has the need to forgive others who truly thought they were doing what was best. I try to comfort myself with that thought, knowing all too well, I have far to go in that regard. I am still on this journey, living and learning. I certainly do not have the answers. I hope just like you, I continue to ask the right questions, even though I may never find the answers.

About the Author: Leo F. Armbrust

Born in Hamilton, Ohio, Leo and his family moved to Hialeah, Florida in 1959. He entered the seminary in 1965 and was ordained a Catholic priest in 1977. During his time in ministry he served as pastoral associate, teacher, counselor, diocesan communications director, and chaplain for sports teams both collegiate and professional. He resigned from active ministry in 2010.

In 2005, Leo devoted all of his energies into the establishment of a facility for homeless youth known as Vita Nova. This organization serves the youth, ages 18-25, transitioning from foster care into independent living. His association with football allowed him to meet and befriend individuals of high net worth. Through their generosity and kindness, he was able to raise more than thirty million dollars to fund this dream.

He has taught on every level of academia and seeks to expand the classroom to include as many as possible. His life experiences, formal education (M.Div., Master of Divinity; M.Th., Master of Theology; M.S.Ed., Master of Education), and thirst for knowledge compelled him to share with others what he has learned.

Leo F. Armbrust is a notary public, a golfer, and open water diver, and a black belt in Tae Kwon Do. His hobbies and interests include cooking, baking, gardening, traveling, reading, writing, and being an avid sports fan.

Readers are welcome to learn more about Leo at his website: www.leoarmbrust.com

www.ingramcontent.com/pod-product-compliance
Lightning Source LLC
Chambersburg PA
CBHW070547090426
42735CB00013B/3100